Practical Strategies for Greatness in Nursing

Drawing on the writings, moral vision, and enduring influence of Florence Nightingale, this book explores timeless principles that are still relevant to nursing today. Fusing historical insight with contemporary theory, it reimagines Nightingale's legacy not as a relic, but as a dynamic guide for present-day practice.

What nursing is, and what it ought to be, has long been the subject of debate. Unlike many other health professions, nursing defies simple categorisation. Its theoretical foundations are wide-ranging, its daily practice often obscured by complexity, and its impact, though essential, frequently overlooked or misunderstood. This inherent ambiguity is part of why the notion of 'greatness' in nursing remains difficult to pin down. *Practical Strategies for Greatness in Nursing: The Nightingale Effect* confronts this issue head-on. Rather than indulging in nostalgia, this book engages critically with the real conditions of modern nursing. It draws on concepts such as 'rebel nurse leadership' and David Graeber's theory of 'bullshit jobs' to challenge the bureaucratisation of care and to advocate for a return to values-led, purpose-driven nursing.

Designed for early-career nurses, students, and aspiring nurse leaders, this accessible book is a motivational resource for enhancing professional identity and impact.

Matthew Wynn is a senior lecturer in adult nursing at Liverpool John Moores University, specialising in wound care, infection control, and the application of digital technologies in healthcare. His academic and clinical experience includes roles in the UK National Health Service and as a commissioned officer in the British Army Reserves. Matthew has contributed to numerous publications and conferences on a range of contemporary clinical, pedagogical, and theoretical issues related to modern nursing practice.

Practical Strategies for Greatness in Nursing
The Nightingale Effect

Matthew Wynn

Routledge
Taylor & Francis Group

LONDON AND NEW YORK

First published 2026
by Routledge
4 Park Square, Milton Park, Abingdon, Oxon OX14 4RN

and by Routledge
605 Third Avenue, New York, NY 10158

Routledge is an imprint of the Taylor & Francis Group, an informa business

British Library Cataloguing-in-Publication Data
A catalogue record for this book is available from the British Library

ISBN: 978-1-041-08612-3 (hbk)
ISBN: 978-1-041-19801-7 (pbk)
ISBN: 978-1-003-64625-9 (ebk)

DOI: 10.4324/9781003646259

Typeset in Times New Roman
by codeMantra

Contents

Foreword

I began my nursing career as a nursing assistant in a hospice. It was there I first saw the true heart of nursing, the compassion, skill, and commitment it takes to care for people at their most vulnerable. I went on to train through Project 2000, which at the time was a new and ambitious approach to nurse education. Even then, I remember feeling a deep sense of frustration with the systems around me. I could see the potential in nursing, but too often it felt constrained by outdated models, siloed thinking, and under-recognised leadership.

That frustration never left me, but it evolved into something far more productive: a mission. In every role I've held since, whether at the bedside, in leadership, or influencing national policy, I've carried with me the belief that nursing must lead, not follow. That we must shape the systems we work in. And that, like Florence Nightingale, we must work through others, building alliances and developing future generations to go further than we ever could alone.

This book captures that spirit brilliantly. It doesn't just recount Florence's legacy; it reclaims her as the revolutionary she truly was. Too often, she's reduced to the "lady with the lamp", a symbol of compassion. But Florence was a radical thinker, a statistician, a strategist, and a communicator of exceptional power. She combined intellectual rigour with the ability to convey complex ideas in both the written and spoken word, skills that allowed her to influence those in power and reshape the healthcare of her time. She didn't separate her analytical mind from her nursing identity; she used one to strengthen the other. And that is the kind of thinking we need today.

What makes this book especially powerful is the way it draws on Nightingale's prolific writing, her ideas, insights, and her many great quotes that have stood the test of time. The author uses these to great effect, expanding on them beautifully to distil ten key lessons for nursing greatness. These lessons are each individually important, but it is their intersectionality that produces the truly great nurse. Not just someone skilled in one area, but someone who can think critically, act compassionately, lead decisively, and influence systems. Importantly, the book makes clear that greatness in nursing is not about hierarchy. Nurses at all levels can embrace these lessons. Greatness is in how we think, act, and lead wherever we are.

Now, as we enter the fourth industrial revolution, driven by technology, AI, and data, we have another opportunity to redefine nursing. I often ask myself: what would Florence do with the tools we now have? She wouldn't just be part of the conversation; she would be shaping it. Leading it. And that's what this book calls us to do.

That vision is at the heart of FutureNurse.uk, the platform I founded to connect nursing with healthtech and drive forward practice innovation. We aim to evolve care by working across professional boundaries, creating new narratives for nursing, and developing technologies that serve the profession – not the other way around. Our work is inspired by the same principles explored in this book: leadership, clarity of purpose, collaboration, and the courage to challenge the status quo.

I only wish I'd had this book at the start of my career. It would have helped me make sense of the challenges I faced and shown me a clearer path to turning frustration into impact, not just for individual patients, but for the systems we work in.

This book is essential reading for anyone in nursing, whether you're just starting out, deep in practice, in training, or in a leadership role. It reminds us not just of what nursing is, but of what it *could be*.

—Professor Natasha Phillips
Founder, FutureNurse.uk
Visiting Professor of Digital Health, University of Salford

Preface

I attribute my success to this: - I never gave or took an excuse. Yes, I do see the difference now between me and other men. When a disaster happens, I act, and they make excuses.[1]

Florence Nightingale to Hilary Bonham Carter 1861

Florence Nightingale, born on May 12, 1820, in Florence, Italy, is celebrated as the foundational philosopher of modern nursing and a pioneering figure in healthcare reform. Renowned for her leadership during the Crimean War, where she drastically reduced death rates by implementing improved sanitation practices, Nightingale's contributions extend beyond her legendary nocturnal rounds to comfort the wounded, earning her the epithet 'The Lady with the Lamp'. Her rigorous statistical advocacy transformed hospital conditions, and her seminal work, 'Notes on Nursing', published in 1859, laid the principles for nursing education and practice. A visionary statistician and social reformer, Nightingale also established the world's first secular nursing school at St. Thomas' Hospital in London, profoundly influencing the professionalisation of nursing and setting standards that have shaped healthcare practices globally. Her reputation among professional and social commentators has undergone significant reappraisal over the years. Initially celebrated as a healthcare pioneer, her legacy has been contested by some who argue that her approach sometimes overshadowed contributions from other nursing figures and underplayed the collaborative nature of healthcare. Critics have also scrutinised her management style and her strict, sometimes autocratic, implementation of hospital reforms. Despite these controversies, her foundational role in modern nursing theory and practice, as well as her statistical innovations in healthcare, remain undisputed. Nightingale's methods and ethos in nursing education have endured, influencing generations and embodying the spirit of the nursing profession. As debates around her legacy continue, she remains, unequivocally, the most well-known and impactful nurse to have ever lived.

In writing this book, I confront a persistent challenge in defining the scope of nursing practice, a dilemma that complicates our understanding of what it means to be a truly 'great' nurse. Florence Nightingale, the founder of modern nursing, herself grappled with these issues, acknowledging in her seminal work, *Notes on Nursing*, that '*the very elements of nursing are all but unknown*'.[2] She further observed that effective nursing should align with the body's natural reparative processes, cautioning that poor nursing practices could hinder rather than support recovery. These reflections underscored her reservations about formalising nursing education, torn between theoretical knowledge and practical training, and the role of medical knowledge within nursing curricula.

Despite the passage of time, these concerns remain markedly relevant today, perhaps even more convoluted than in Nightingale's era. Throughout the 20th century, significant efforts were made to establish a unified theory of nursing, yet these theories have struggled to make a meaningful impact on the profession beyond as the foci for primarily academic, not clinical, work.[3] Nightingale herself worried about the medical profession's encroachment into nursing, fearing it might detract from the pursuit of a distinct nursing knowledge, a concern that echoes through the ages as contemporary nursing increasingly veers towards what some scholars describe as the 'medicalisation of nursing'.[4] These challenges, whilst troublesome from the perspective of educators and policymakers, and arguably contributory in the ongoing lack of understanding around the true nature of nursing work among the public, do have their upsides. Specifically, the profession's flexibility and adaptability enable it to address problems across the broad field of healthcare. As we shall see, the lessons from Nightingale do not point towards specific sources of knowledge or clinical skills per se, to achieve greatness in nursing.

The under-recognition of nurses and their contributions is another theme this book addresses. Nurses may feel their work is overshadowed by societal perceptions or by the medical field, a sentiment likely exacerbated by the ways in which nurses publicise and conduct their work. Drawing from Nightingale's example, this book seeks to support the elevation and visibility and understanding of nursing's unique impact, via an examination of the means with which Nightingale achieved this. This work is not intended as a biographical account of Nightingale, nor does it aim to introduce new information about her life or legacy. It also doesn't intend to be a hagiography; Nightingale was certainly an imperfect character like all people, however she undoubtedly remains the most well-known and perhaps impactful nurse that ever lived. Accordingly, reflective analysis aimed at distilling what modern nurses might learn from Nightingale to achieve recognition and impact comparable to hers arguably remains a worthwhile endeavour. Where the mythology surrounding her life is a consequence of factors beyond her direct control, or where there are negative lessons, these are duly acknowledged. Ultimately, this book is to support development of nurses work towards achieving what I term the '*Nightingale Effect*',* an enduring impact on professional affairs in

---

* Nothing to do with falling in love or falling into nursing. This is about rising to it.

healthcare, and public and political perceptions of nursing for the benefit of humanity.

To frame these discussions, I draw heavily on the excellent biographical work by Mark Bostridge[5] and Lynn McDonald,[6,7] alongside Nightingale's own extensive writings to understand her character and the nature of her work. The reflections on contemporary challenges in the nursing profession are considered through the lens of Nightingale's philosophies and the potential for Nightingalean efforts in today's nursing landscape. It is worth remarking upon however, the shear volume of writing and material associated with Nightingale generated during her lifetime. The fact she attained fame early in her life has likely also increased the quantity of this which has been preserved and remains accessible, with new original source material being published even a century after her death. As such, investigations into her life and work could fuel a lifetime worth of research. This work reflects only what I can usefully distil into a concise book, aimed principally at contemporary nurses.

While Florence Nightingale is central to this analysis, it's important to clarify why other historical figures in nursing, such as Mary Seacole, are not comparably featured. Seacole has often been celebrated for her contributions to nursing, sometimes referred to as the 'Black Nightingale'. These comparisons, however, as noted by Mark Bostridge, *'do not belong in the realm of serious history'*[5] due to the significantly different roles and contributions each made within the field of healthcare during their lifetimes. Furthermore, Lynn McDonald's work, 'Mary Seacole: The Making of the Myth',[8] provides an in-depth exploration of how Seacole's legacy has been constructed and sometimes misconstrued over time. It bears noting that my first academic position was based in the Mary Seacole Building at the University of Salford, a naming that indicates the respect and recognition afforded to Seacole in the UK and beyond. However, it is a disservice to both Nightingale and Seacole to conflate their historical impacts or to misrepresent their contributions to nursing; it is also worth considering that Seacole never considered herself a nurse but instead a 'doctress'. By focusing exclusively on Nightingale in this book, I aim to explore her specific philosophies and strategies without diluting the narrative with less directly comparable figures. This focused approach allows us to glean the most relevant lessons from Nightingale's work, applying them to contemporary nursing challenges while respecting the unique and separate legacy of Mary Seacole.

This book is structured around ten pivotal lessons from Nightingale's work in nursing. This includes not just exploration of Nightingales direct teachings, but also analysis on her actions. In some cases, the lessons she gave her nurses were at odds with the behaviours she demonstrated themselves, as will be seen, these may well have had a significant influence on the reputation which she established for herself.

Each chapter not only explores these lessons, but also offers practical, actionable advice alongside reflective questions designed to support their integration into contemporary nursing practice. Through this exploration, the book aims to inspire nurses to strive to achieve the Nightingale effect, to make a lasting impact on their profession and, more importantly, the people they care for.

References

1. Cook, E. T. (1913). *The Life of Florence Nightingale* (Vol. 1, p.506). Macmillan and Company. (Original letter from Florence Nightingale to Miss H. Bonham Carter dated 1861). https://hdl.handle.net/2027/uc2.ark:/13960/t9h421p1x?urlappend=%3Bseq=54
2. Nightingale, F. *Notes on Nursing.* Lippincott Williams & Wilkins. [Original work published 1859]. https://digital.library.upenn.edu/women/nightingale/nursing/nursing.html
3. Thorne, S. (2023). On the contribution of the nursing theorists. In *Routledge Handbook of Philosophy and Nursing* (1st ed., p. 11). Routledge.
4. McCarthy, M. P., & Jones, J. S. (2019). The medicalization of nursing: The loss of a discipline's unique identity. *International Journal for Human Caring,* 23(1), 101–108. https://doi.org/10.20467/1091-5710.23.1.101
5. Bostridge, M. (2008). Florence Nightingale: *The Woman and Her Legend* (p.278). Penguin UK.
6. McDonald, L. Ed. Nightingale, F. *The Collected Works of Florence Nightingale.* https://cwfn.uoguelph.ca/short-papers-excerpts/
7. McDonald, L. (2017). *Florence Nightingale: A Very Brief History.* SPCK.
8. McDonald, L. (2017). *Mary Seacole: The Making of the* Myth Iguana.

Acknowledgements

The list of individuals, nurses and otherwise, who have contributed to the thinking and reflections that led to this book is far too long to fit within these pages. However, there are some to whom I must offer particular thanks. First, my wife Lizzie: an inspiringly skilled nurse and the greatest supporter of my work. This project (along with many others) would not have been possible without her. To my colleague Natasha Phillips, a pioneer of digital nursing and a fellow admirer of Nightingale, who not only contributed the foreword to this book, but also helped shape my thinking around the profession, particularly in the digital age.

Finally, to Sarah Watmough, who so generously took the time to proofread the manuscript. Any errors in the book, of course, remain entirely my own.

Reconceptualising nursing greatness

A critical lens on Florence Nightingale's legacy

'Greatness' is an elusive concept in nursing* but its importance cannot be over-stated. It represents something to strive for, a sense of purpose that goes beyond the day-to-day tasks and reaches into the very heart of what it means to care for others. Achieving greatness in nursing doesn't just elevate an individual; it raises the standard for the entire profession. It reflects meta-leadership, where one nurse's actions ripple across the healthcare landscape, improving systems, policies, and practices for the benefit of countless patients. A pursuit of greatness may make a nursing career more fulfilling, offering a sense of personal and professional achievement that goes beyond simple job satisfaction. However, the path to greatness in nursing is uniquely challenging and seldom talked about. Unlike in medicine, where success is often measured in clear tangible outcomes like new surgical achievements or improvements in diagnostic precision, nursing outcomes are often harder to quantify. A surgeon may be recognised world-wide for developing a breakthrough procedure, but a nurse's greatness is often experienced at a deeply personal level, in quiet moments of care that are rarely publicised. Even among nursing scholars, there's no consensus on a single definition of nursing that captures the vast range of roles and responsibilities nurses take on. The common thread, however, is the betterment of patients' health and well-being. Nurses, unlike many doctors, also rarely work fully independently. Their efforts are often absorbed into the broader tapestry of the healthcare team, making individual recognition difficult. While the complexity of performing surgery is easily recognised, the less visible but equally vital work of nurses often goes unheralded. Yet, Florence Nightingale showed us the profound power a single nurse can have in transforming healthcare systems. Her work during the Crimean War demonstrated for the first time the significant and lasting impact that individuals can have.

Yet, the pursuit of greatness in nursing today faces unprecedented challenges. The healthcare landscape has become more complex. Nurses are working in

---

* The term 'greatness' is used, for lack of a better word, to encapsulate the transformative impact and enduring legacy of Florence Nightingale's nursing principles, referred to also as the 'Nightingale effect'.

DOI: 10.4324/9781003646259-1

a system that often prioritises efficiency and productivity over patient-centred care, placing greater pressure on individual practitioners. The demands of the profession, rising patient caseloads, technological advancements, regulatory hurdles, and global pandemics, can make the notion of 'greatness' seem out of reach, or at best a secondary concern to the immediate tasks involved in providing a basic level of care. However, it is precisely during these difficult times that the pursuit of greatness becomes even more critical. Nurses who can rise above the challenges of modern healthcare, by advocating for their patients, engaging with new technologies without losing their humanness, and consistently striving for excellence, are those who will continue to transform the profession. This book is not about what it means to be a good nurse; it is about what it might mean to be a *great* nurse. It is within the capabilities of all nurses to be good, to care effectively for the patients whose care they are charged with. This is a perfectly respectable status to attain and undoubtedly invaluable to society.[†] One does not have to be an Olympic champion to be among the best athletes in the world. However, there are those who wish to go beyond 'goodness' to achieve the status of *greatness*, to become international leaders in the profession, just like Nightingale. This book is a guide to those nurses. The guidance contained within may be difficult to put into practice, but this is precisely the reason why greatness is so rare.

Nursing as a calling

Perhaps the first step to nursing greatness is to consider the question of why become a nurse in the first place? Nursing is in some cases thought of as more than a career; it was considered by Nightingale to be a calling. This concept of 'calling' is not without its critics. In modern nursing discourse, the idea of a 'calling' has been debated, with some arguing that it risks reinforcing outdated perceptions of nursing as a self-sacrificial or subordinate profession. For Nightingale however, to be a nurse requires not just skill and knowledge but a deep sense of moral duty. Florence Nightingale, often regarded as the founder of modern professional nursing, embodied this calling in everything she did. Born into a wealthy British family, she defied societal expectations by choosing to devote her life to caring for the sick. Driven by her strong Christian faith, she believed that her work was a form of service to God,

> I do, forgetting those things which are behind, and reaching forth unto those things which are before, I press toward the mark for the prize of the high calling of God in Christ Jesus; and what higher "calling" can we have that Nursing?[1]
>
> Nightingale – Lecture to her nurses 1872

---

† I vividly remember the profound pride I felt after completing demanding 12-hour shifts as a staff nurse, knowing the difference I had made to individual patients, even as I walked back to my apartment exhausted, dehydrated, and aware that I would return to the ward in less than 12 hours.

Her strong sense of duty, founded in her Christian faith, laid the foundation for nursing as a profession, one that requires both intellectual and emotional investment. However, greatness in nursing does not require faith in a religious sense. It requires a shared commitment to the core values of nursing: the inherent dignity, worth, and sanctity of human life. These values can be derived from diverse sources, whether religious traditions, secular humanism, or a deeply personal conviction in the importance of compassionate care. Unusually for the time, Nightingale did advocate for strictly secular training schools for nursing. This was perhaps partly due to the inherent divisiveness of sectarian religious activities, an issue which formed the focus of media attention on her during her lifetime; but also due to her beliefs that prayer was a misdirection of human energy, and that achievement of her religious purposes could be achieved only via concrete action to improve the world.

While some may prefer not to frame nursing as a 'calling', this term is understood here to recognise the profound sense of responsibility, ethical commitment, and dedication that nursing demands, which Nightingale undoubtedly recognised. It is critical to also emphasise that nursing is a highly skilled profession that requires appropriate recognition, remuneration, and resources. Calling and professionalism are arguably not mutually exclusive; they complement each other to create the foundation of great nursing practice. Achieving greatness as a nurse includes recognising one's limits and prioritising self-care. Florence Nightingale's tireless dedication is inspirational, but it should not be misinterpreted as a call to work oneself to exhaustion. To truly answer the 'calling' of nursing, one must balance professional commitment with personal well-being to sustain a career in this demanding yet profoundly rewarding field. Nightingale would likely have agreed, during her time in Scutari, she would reportedly often work for 20 hours at a time, largely disregarding her own health. She did, however, take a weekly walk on Sundays to relax in a vapour bath.[2] In modern nursing, honouring both dedication and self-preservation is essential to upholding the spirit of Nightingale's legacy.

Contemporary philosophers of nursing have highlighted the pragmatic challenges with dwelling on these moral components to nursing.[3] In contemporary nurse education, competencies often include direct references to the demonstration of 'compassion', 'courage', 'humility', and 'empathy'. These are, it is argued, both inherently unmeasurable and also often not reflected in the real-world practices of many nurses. It is also argued that they reflect a gendered sacrificial expectation of nurses, perpetuating outdated views of nursing as a primarily feminine, altruistic vocation, potentially overshadowing the clinical expertise and professional autonomy that ought to characterise contemporary nursing practice.[‡] However, the concept of a calling, often tied

---

‡ For a detailed exploration of the persistent issues related to gender in nursing, refer to Davies, C. (1995). *Gender and the Professional Predicament in Nursing*. Buckingham, England: Open University Press. Although published over three decades ago, the insights presented in this work remain strikingly relevant to contemporary discussions on gender dynamics within the nursing profession.

to personal and financial sacrifice, is arguably not unique to nursing but can be seen across various fields, particularly in entrepreneurship. Entrepreneurs frequently discuss the need to make substantial sacrifices to achieve success. In nursing, however, this sacrifice is compounded by a moral dimension, the belief in the inherent goodness of sacrificing for the health and well-being of others. This aspect of nursing's calling elevates it beyond mere occupational dedication, infusing it with a profound ethical and humanitarian commitment which is often at odds with business-oriented healthcare systems which do not place great financial value on such sacrifices for individuals.

Despite the inspirational power of such a calling, it presents a paradox for modern nursing education and practice. The inherent nature of motivation, deeply personal and not easily alterable, suggests that while the historical example of Florence Nightingale's driven pursuit might inspire, it is not necessarily a template that can be directly applied or taught in contemporary settings. Anne Marie Rafferty and Rosemary Wall suggest that '*she probably never felt of duty: the clock was ticking, and she might die before her work was done*'.[4] Nightingale's success, fuelled by a seemingly unyielding drive and a unique set of circumstances, resulted in significant advancements in healthcare and established a lasting legacy. However, the emphasis on such extraordinary levels of dedication risks setting an unsustainable standard for modern nurses. Recognising the dual demands of calling and professionalism within nursing is crucial. While the historical context of nursing as a calling can offer valuable lessons in dedication and ethical practice, it is essential to balance these with a realistic appreciation of the professional and personal boundaries necessary for sustaining a healthy and productive career in nursing. Greatness in nursing is likely to require a personal investment in one's own professional development that extends beyond the standard 9-to-5 schedule, but, crucially, as this chapter argues, such ambition must be tempered with an ongoing commitment to balance, to ensure that personal development remains empowering rather than exploitative. Acknowledging this balance can help redefine nursing's calling for the 21st century, ensuring it supports both the personal well-being of nurses and their professional excellence without requiring nurses to martyr themselves to their profession.

The legacy of Florence Nightingale

The legacy of Florence Nightingale continues to influence nursing today and remains the subject of books examining her influence on modern healthcare.[5,6] She took ownership of problems that others ignored, often working against the odds to improve conditions in hospitals and create lasting change. When she arrived in Crimea, the hospital was a death trap: filthy, overcrowded, and understaffed. Nightingale revolutionised the system, implementing sanitation practices that dramatically reduced mortality rates. She did all of this while battling opposition from medical professionals and military authorities who, in some instances, resisted her reforms. Her relentless focus on patient outcomes, regardless of the obstacles, serves as a powerful example for nurses today. Indeed, her name still evokes a sense of security and order in chaotic situations. In the UK, the field hospitals deployed rapidly following the outbreak of the COVID-19 virus in 2020 were named 'Nightingale Hospitals'. This is testament to not only her lasting imprint on the nursing profession, but of the impact she remains to have on the population at large. Indeed, Nightingale, at least at the time of writing and as far as the author is aware, is the only nurse to have an entire museum dedicated to her, situated on the south bank of the river Thames in London.

Nightingale also understood the importance of supporting others. She didn't just make changes herself, she developed others around her, ensuring that her reforms would continue long after she was gone. This spirit of mentorship and development is central to nursing leadership today. Whether you are guiding new nurses or driving change within your team, the principles Nightingale laid down – courage, innovation, and unwavering dedication to patient care – are as essential now as they were in her time. It is important to acknowledge, however, that Nightingale did have certain privileges that may have contributed to her prominence as a great historical figure. Born into an upper-middle-class British family, Nightingale had access to wealth, education, and social influence, advantages that most women, let alone nurses, of her time did not possess. Her background allowed her to move in elite circles, converse with influential policymakers, and access resources that many of her peers couldn't dream of. This, no doubt, played a role in amplifying her efforts and ensuring her place in history.

However, it would be a mistake to attribute Nightingale's greatness solely to her social standing. In fact, she actively resisted the expectations placed on her by her family and society. Nursing in the 19th century was seen as a lowly profession, unfit for a woman of her status. Her family wanted her to marry well and live a life of comfort, but Nightingale had a calling for nursing that she could not ignore, shunning societal norms and her family's wishes. This act of defiance was, perhaps, the first sign of the greatness that would manifest in her groundbreaking work. Nightingale's wealth and connections could have provided her with a life of ease, yet they did not hand her the courage, tenacity, and vision that marked her accomplishments. Money alone does not create moral leadership, nor does it inspire someone to revolutionise healthcare practices, establish a nursing school, or advocate tirelessly for public health reforms internationally. Nightingale's commitment to nursing was not just a product of her privilege, it was driven by a deep sense of purpose and moral conviction. As Laurence Housemen observed within his essay on Nightingale within an edited collection on 'The Great Victorians':

> …Though her popularity greatly lightened her task, and made much that she did possible, which might otherwise have remained impossible, it is still probably true that hers was the most towering ability, as it was surely the most unusual in kind…[7]

Her choice to go against the grain and pursue nursing, despite its low social standing, reveals some of the intrinsic qualities that made her memorable: perseverance, empathy, and a relentless drive to improve the world around her. These are the traits that transcend time and social status, and they are lessons from which we can all learn, regardless of our own backgrounds. Nightingale's life is a reminder that greatness is not about where you come from, but how you choose to navigate your circumstances and the lasting impact you create, often against considerable odds and when there are numerous reasons to give up.

References

1   Nightingale, F. (1915). *Nightingale to Her Nurses: A Selection from Miss Nightingale's Addresses to Probationers and Nurses of the Nightingale School at St Thomas's Hospital* (p. 4). Macmillan and Co. Limited.
2   Bostridge, M. (2008). *Florence Nightingale: The Woman and Her Legend* (p. 246). Penguin.
3   Drevdahl, D. J., & Canales, M. K. (2023). Nursing's endless pursuit of professionalization. In Martin Lipscomb (Ed.), *Routledge Handbook of Philosophy and Nursing* (pp. 215–226). Routledge. https://doi.org/10.4324/9781003427407-26
4   Nelson, S., & Rafferty, A. M. (Eds.). (2010). *Notes on Nightingale: The Influence and Legacy of a Nursing Icon* (p. 140). ILR Press.
5   Rafferty, A. M., & Wall, B. (2010). An icon and iconoclast for today. In S. Nelson & A. M. Rafferty (Eds.), *Notes on Nightingale: The Influence and Legacy of a Nursing Icon* (pp. 130–141). ILR Press.
6   McDonald, L. (2017). *Florence Nightingale, Nursing, and Health Care Today.* Springer.
7   Houseman in Massingham, H. J., & Massingham, H. (1937). *The Great Victorians* (p. 364). Penguin Books. http://localhost:8080/jspui/handle/123456789/2319

1 Advocating for vulnerable patients

Be the Guardian of the Silent

Advocacy in a healthcare context refers to the act of supporting or arguing in favour of a specific cause, policy, or individual's rights within the health system. It involves promoting and protecting the interests of patients by ensuring they receive appropriate care, respect, and information to make informed decisions about their treatment. Advocacy aims to empower patients, address inequalities, and improve health outcomes by actively intervening, educating, and influencing healthcare practices and policies on behalf of those who may not have the voice or resources to do so themselves.

Florence Nightingale's legacy is built not only on her groundbreaking work in nursing but also on her unyielding commitment to advocacy within both healthcare and society more broadly.* In an era where nurses were typically expected to follow the orders of doctors and military authorities without question, Nightingale dared to challenge the status quo. She believed that the health, dignity, and well-being of her patients came first, and she wasn't afraid to speak up, even when it meant clashing with those in power. Providing a voice for the less fortunate was a frequent feature of Nightingales work. At a time where racism was the norm, she promoted liberal perspectives and alongside her family was ardently anti-slavery. [1] Her later work included research into the conditions of indigenous communities in Australian, Sri Lanka, South Africa, and Canada.[2] In the 1860s, the introduction of Contagious Diseases Legislation to control the spread of venereal disease within the Army and Navy, requiring undignified registration and invasive internal examinations of prostitutes to identify 'unclean' women resulted in advocacy efforts from Nightingale.[3] She collected data which demonstrated that this approach to preventing the spread of infection was flawed and promoted the argument that

---

* A notable example of her advocacy is reflected in her lesser-known work, 'Cassandra', which critiques the restrictions placed on women of her time, expressing her frustration over the lack of meaningful work available to women and advocating for greater female participation in professional roles. A situation which was to partly be alleviated by the foundation of the Nightingale school of nursing.

DOI: 10.4324/9781003646259-2

facilitating better living conditions for the soldiers may reduce their reliance on 'vice' thereby advocating simultaneously for the women and the soldiers.[4] Publication of her appeals subsequently gained wide support.

When she was superintendent at the Harley Street Establishment for Gentle-Women during illness, against considerable opposition in allowing patients from a variety of religious backgrounds to be admitted.[5] It is worth considering in this case, however, that her status as a 'lady' may have influenced the decision made by the hospital committee to yield to her demands. However, the emphasis she placed on this particular issue was perhaps not only a consequence of her belief in the inherent sanctity of human dignity, but also due to her forward-thinking political strategy for the nursing profession. She was aware of the sectarian issues inherent in British society and that nurses may be seen to be fulfilling a primarily religious mission. This issue was to reappear later when she was directly ordered to ensure balance in the religious makeup of her nursing staff in the Crimea to ensure there was no perception that nurses were actively seeking to convert wounded soldiers to Catholicism.[6] In advocating in this way, Nightingale not only ensured equitable access to care for her patients but also ensured that perceptions of her nursing aims were not contaminated by the sectarian disputes of the contemporary social culture.

To be a relentless advocate for patients means taking ownership of their care and acting as their voice when they cannot speak for themselves. It also means having the skill and criticality to identify when a system, policy, or practice is putting patients at risk and taking action to protect their rights, safety, and dignity. Nightingale's approach to advocacy teaches us that greatness in nursing lies in the *willingness* to challenge authority and champion what is right for the patient.

Nightingale's advocacy: clashing with authority in the Crimean War (1854–1856)

When Florence Nightingale arrived at the British military hospital in Scutari in 1854, she was confronted with deplorable conditions that were leading to high mortality rates among soldiers. Nightingale recognised that the hospital itself was killing the soldiers, and she immediately took it upon herself to advocate for their well-being.

Nightingale faced stiff resistance from both military leaders and the medical establishment. At the time, military authorities prioritised logistics and military protocols over patient care, and many doctors were dismissive of her concerns. Despite this opposition, Nightingale was determined to advocate for the soldiers. Her refusal to back down in the face of powerful opposition is a hallmark of her relentless advocacy. Nightingale's efforts eventually paid off. She secured better supplies, improved sanitation, and implemented protocols that dramatically reduced the death rate in military hospitals. By the end of her first winter at Scutari, the mortality rate had dropped from 42% to 2%. This monumental shift wasn't just the result of medical care; it was the product of Nightingale's tireless advocacy, which pushed the boundaries of what was expected from a nurse at the time. Moreover, her personal commitment to the soldiers and their families was profound. Nightingale not only personally funded care[7] for bereaved families but also wrote them personal letters, informing the families of what had happened to their sons; marking a significant moment as it was the first time such communications came from an official source.[7] This level of personal involvement was virtually unheard of at the time due to the low value placed on the concerns of ordinary soldiers. This reflects her unique approach to nursing and healthcare and is consistent with the 'person-centred' approaches to nursing advocated for today.

Legal and ethical dimensions of advocacy

Nurses are now bound by professional codes of ethics that emphasise the importance of patient advocacy. This began in earnest in the 1970s, when the International Council of Nursing first utilised the term, a development that helped establish advocacy as a defining responsibility of the profession.[8] Nursing codes of ethics typically state that nurses must act to safeguard the health, safety, and rights of patients, even when this requires confronting institutional or societal barriers. This encourages nurses to intervene when patient care is compromised, whether due to poor staffing, inadequate resources, or unethical policies.

Advocacy also involves protecting patients' legal rights. Due to unique proximity to patients, nurses are often the first to identify when a patient's rights are being violated, whether in terms of consent, confidentiality, or treatment options. In many cases, it is considered the nurse's responsibility to ensure that patients understand their rights and are given the opportunity to make informed decisions about their care. This might involve advocating for a patient's right to refuse treatment, ensuring they have access to necessary medical information, or intervening when their care is mismanaged. In these situations, nurses act as the frontline defenders of patient autonomy and dignity.

Overcoming barriers to advocacy

Advocating for patients is not without its challenges. Nurses, like Nightingale, often face resistance from those in positions of power. Contemporary studies of advocacy highlight many of these barriers including a lack of support from colleagues, organisational resistance, limited time, legal support, anticipated negative outcomes, ineffective communication, and interpersonal relationships among many others.[9] Other authors have sought to synthesise the characteristics that make for effective nurse advocates identifying five key approaches.[10]

1 *Understanding the context*

As in Nightingales time, the socio-political influences on the nursing profession are ever-present. Whilst sectarian conflicts have largely dissipated in most industrialised countries, the political and cultural influences on nursing continue to create challenges that affect how nursing care is delivered and how nurses advocate for their patients. For instance, the introduction of digital health records and telemedicine requires nurses to adapt rapidly, ensuring they safeguard patient from digital harms, now referred to as 'e-iatrogenesis'.[11] Additionally, global health emergencies, such as the COVID-19 pandemic, have underscored the need for nurses to be vocal advocates for both resource allocation and public health strategies, highlighting the ongoing importance of understanding and responding to the socio-political dimensions of healthcare. Finally, the gendered nature of nursing undoubtedly continues to play a role in professional dynamics in addition to public and political perceptions. Crucially, a robust contextual awareness in nursing requires careful reflection on the way that nurses are perceived by those outside the profession, including by political authorities. These perceptions may be incongruent with the professional identity desired by nursing authorities or individual nurses. To navigate the complexities of modern healthcare, nurses must not only master clinical skills but also develop a critical consciousness of the broader forces that shape their practice and public image. This consciousness may in turn, guide more effective advocacy, guiding actions which accurately consider context.

2 *Problem solving*

Understanding the root of the problem is often the key to achieving successful advocacy outcomes. In the case of Nightingales efforts to eliminate undignified internal examinations of women and address the lack of available pastimes for the soldiers, she understood that it was the transmission of venereal disease which was the key issue of interest to policymakers. Rather than appealing to emotion via a moral argument, she instead collected clear data on rates of venereal disease to indicate the value of this approach. This ultimately proved persuasive to some key decision-makers at the time. Nurses today should consider how their advocacy arguments may be made most persuasively using data and evidence. Whilst ethics may initiate action, as Nightingale demonstrated, rhetorical impact is the key to success in advocacy.

3   *Build relationships*
    Understanding who the key stakeholders are is key to understanding how to advocate for change. Political skills are not emphasised in contemporary nursing education. However, Nightingale evidently understood this and frequently worked through others to achieve her aims. This is an issue which is returned to later in Chapter 6.

4   Develop communication skills
    The ability to appreciate context and identify problems, including via the collection and analysis of data is unlikely to influence key decision-makers without any ability to communicate. Nightingale wrote prolifically throughout her lifetime. This included extensive surveying and publicising data related to the living conditions and healthcare in India, a country she had never even visited.[12] The success of her advocacy work in this context continues to have a lasting impact in India. In a 2025 article in the Indian Express discussing Nightingale's legacy and ongoing influence on modern healthcare, it is argued that *'She wielded science like a poet and compassion like a warrior, redefining health as a right, not a privilege. For an Indian audience, her lamp isn't a relic; it's a flare in the dark of today's disparities'.*[13]

5   Influence
    Credibility and trustworthiness are critical when seeking to influence others. Whilst nursing is often reported to be the most trustworthy profession[14] it is not a given that this means nurses are listened to when advocating for their patients or themselves. Credibility is gained by demonstrating awareness of context, insight into the problem, clear and effective collaboration with other key stakeholders and the ability to coherently communicate the solution to problems using appropriate and sufficient evidence.

Arguably, the challenges of patient advocacy are no different today than they were in Nightingale's time, nor are the solutions any more challenging, as Rafferty and Wall argue:

> We need Nightingales for the twenty-first century providing the moral and scientific leadership necessary to advocate for patients using best evidence to deliver effective, safe and compassionate care…The continuous need to improve the quality of healthcare is a constant quest of all health systems but that quest comes first and foremost from the individual.[15]

Without taking these factors into account, as Nightingale undoubtedly did, within advocacy efforts, the results may be frustrated and not result in sustained change.

Key lessons for modern nurses to achieve the Nightingale Effect

- Advocacy is crucial, upholding and championing the interests of patients and nurses is a core responsibility in nursing.
- Challenge practices that harm patient care by demonstrating *both* moral courage and intellectual rigor.
- Use data strategically to identify what is necessary to influence policy and practice effectively.
- Build strategic relationships by engaging with key stakeholders, including those unfamiliar, to support your advocacy goals.
- Understand the socio-political contexts that influence nursing which will differ between settings.
- Prioritise credibility by enhancing your advocacy with strong written and verbal communication skills.

Reflective questions to consider to help you to advocate for people under your care:

1 Would I like myself or my family to be treated in the system I work within?
2 *Who* might be able to help me to improve the care we provide?
3 What are the socio-political influences on nursing in my context and how might this influence my approach to advocacy?

References

1 McDonald, L. *Florence Nightingale: A Leading Anti-Racist*. https://nightingalesociety.com/papers/florence-nightingale-a-leading-anti-racist/

2 Nightingale, F. (2004). Sanitary statistics of native colonial schools and hospitals. In McDonald, L. (Ed.), *Florence Nightingale on Public Health Care* (pp. 168–183). Wilfrid Laurier University Press.

3 Bostridge, M. (2008). *Florence Nightingale: The Woman and Her Legend* (p. 405). Penguin.

4 Nightingale, F. (1862). *Note on the Supposed Protection Afforded Against Venereal Diseases, by Recognizing Prostitution and Putting It under Police Regulation.* Privately printed.

5 Bostridge, M. (2008). *Florence Nightingale: The Woman and Her Legend* (p. 189). Penguin.

6 Paradis, M. R., Hart, E. M., & O'Brien, M. J. (2017). The sisters of Mercy in the Crimean War: Lessons for Catholic health care. *The Linacre Quarterly*, 84(1), 29–43. https://doi.org/10.1080/00243639.2016.1277877

7 Bostridge, M. (2008). *Florence Nightingale: The Woman and Her Legend* (pp. 69, 284). Penguin.
8 Selanders, L., & Crane, P. (2012, January 31). The voice of Florence Nightingale on advocacy. *OJIN: The Online Journal of Issues in Nursing*, 17(1), Manuscript 1.
9 Nsiah, C., Siakwa, M., & Ninnoni, J. P. K. (2020). Barriers to practicing patient advocacy in healthcare setting. *Nursing Open*, 7, 650–659. https://doi.org/10.1002/nop2.436
10 Madigan, E. A., McWhirter, E., Westwood, G., Oshikanlu, R., Iregi, Z. M., Nyika, M., & Bayuo, J. (2023). Nurses finding a global voice by becoming influential leaders through advocacy. *Clinics in Integrated Care*, 20, 100165. Elsevier BV. https://doi.org/10.1016/j.intcar.2023.100165
11 Weiner, J. P., Kfuri, T., Chan, K., & Fowles, J. B. (2007). "e-Iatrogenesis": The most critical unintended consequence of CPOE and other HIT. *Journal of the American Medical Informatics Association: JAMIA*, 14(3), 387–389. https://doi.org/10.1197/jamia.M2338
12 Hays, J. C. (1989). Florence Nightingale and the India sanitary reforms. *Public Health Nursing*, 6(3), 152–154. https://doi.org/10.1111/j.1525-1446.1989.tb00589.x
13 Patel, M. (2025). How Florence Nightingale revolutionised sanitation in India without setting foot in the subcontinent. https://indianexpress.com/article/research/how-florence-nightingale-revolutionised-sanitation-in-india-without-setting-foot-in-the-subcontinent-9873924/
14 American Nurses Association. (2024). America's most trusted: Nurses continue to rank the highest. https://www.nursingworld.org/news/news-releases/2024/americas-most-trusted-nurses-continue-to-rank-the-highest/
15 Rafferty, A. M., & Wall, B. (2010). An icon and iconoclast for today. In Nelson, S., & Rafferty, A. M. (Eds.), *Notes on Nightingale: The Influence and Legacy of a Nursing Icon* (p. 140). ILR Press.

2 Driving systemic healthcare improvements

Heal the System, Not Just the Wound

Florence Nightingale recognised that the root cause of many preventable deaths lay not in the quality of care given at the bedside, but in the broken structures surrounding patient care. Nightingale's focus on systemic reform, changing hospital conditions, advocating for better sanitation, and collecting data to drive decision-making set her apart and created a legacy that continues to guide nursing practice today. Crucially, her disdain for inefficient care and 'red tape' are well known and frequently appear in her writings throughout her career. Rather than simply addressing symptoms, Nightingale treated the hospital as a system in need of intervention. She wrote in the preface of her famous text 'Notes on Hospitals', *'The first requirement in a hospital is that it should do the sick no harm'.*[1]

For Nightingale, this meant focusing on sanitation, ventilation, and proper nutrition, she recognised the dire implications for poorly managed hospital infrastructure and inappropriately utilised human resources. She was keenly aware of the impacts of the organisation of work on the outcomes achievable by healthcare services. In a talk delivered by Nightingale on Army sanitary administration in 1862, she provides the following wisdom:

> The lesson which these reforms teach is that the real foundation of War Office efficiency is to be laid in the efficient working of each Department:- in simplifying procedure - abolishing all divided responsibility - clearly defining the duties of each Officer - in giving direct responsibility to each head of a Department - and, lastly, in placing all the Departmental heads in direct communication with the Secretary of State.[2]

Crucially, role clarity and purpose were identified as key components of a successful healthcare service. This lesson appears to have been largely forgotten in contemporary nursing, however. In Nightingales time, there were no professional regulators of nursing, national clinical nursing policies, established quality standards, and clinical guidelines to be implemented and audited, among many other features of modern healthcare which lend themselves to increasing bureaucratic infrastructure. The issues created by

DOI: 10.4324/9781003646259-3

inefficient services were recognised by the British Governments Department of Health and Social Care (DHSC) in 2020 when they launched a call for evidence to help identify, and therefore reduce, unnecessary bureaucracy.[3] This work identified the most common sources of inefficiency, identifying time consuming procurement processes, duplicative data requests, overly complex regulation, excessive appraisals and mandatory training, poor information management and out of date prescriptive legislation as key factors. The DHSC report indicated that up to a third of community-based clinicians time per working year is spent on administration and patient coordination. These issues would no doubt have exercised Nightingale, who stated in a section on 'petty management' in her Notes on Nursing that nurses should '... *arrange so as that no minute and no hour shall be for her patient without the essentials of her nursing'.*[4] However, as the DHSC do rightly argue, not all bureaucratic work is avoidable and new processes and technologies, namely digital technology and artificial intelligence which may facilitate Nightingale's vision of undisrupted access to nursing care (this is discussed in more depth in Chapter 10). However, whilst process issues and 'red tape' are clearly a source of much inefficiency, Nightingale touched on a more pernicious source of ineffectiveness in her writings, namely that of issues in role definitions. This issue was most thoroughly explored by David Graeber in his thesis on 'bullshit jobs', detailed in his 2018 book of the same name.[5]

Notes on bullshit

Graeber's theory suggests that much work in modern developed societies is pointless, unnecessary, or pernicious. This situation has occurred despite the increasing automation of jobs as per the expectations of a post-industrial revolution society where less time was spent working, and more on enjoying life. Consequences of this proliferation of pointless work are posited as being a form of psychological violence. Nightingale herself was keen to avoid taking on more nurses than she felt was strictly necessary, a perhaps alien concept to modern nurses. In a letter to Sidney Herbert (secretary at war during Nightingale's time in the Crimea), she complained about an incoming party of nurses sent to her hospitals without her requesting them:

> I am willing to bear the evil of governing (& preventing from doing mischief) the non-efficient or scheming majority, which is my great difficulty & most wearing-out labour - because I acknowledge the moral effect produced, which could not have been produced by smaller numbers. But I am not willing to encounter the crowding greater numbers to exhaust our powers & make us useless & incapable. by wasting our time & nervous energy...[6]
>
> Nightingale to Herbert 1854

Nightingale evidently recognised the significance of quality and the ability to manage resources, rather than focussing primarily on quantity. It was argued at the time however, that the presence of a greater number of nurses may provide better publicity for the governments nursing mission.[7] While this political aim is understandable, it bore little relation to the actual needs of nursing care on the ground. As Nightingale's correspondence highlights, the increased numbers risked creating further problems that could undermine the core objectives of her mission.

This tension between genuine need and political display in Nightingale's experience reflects a broader problem later theorised by David Graeber. In his work on 'bullshit jobs', Graeber argues that unnecessary work can take several distinct forms. These include 'flunkies', who exist primarily to make their superiors appear more important; 'goons', who act to manipulate public perceptions for their employers' benefit; 'duct tapers', who provide short-term fixes for systemic problems; 'box tickers', who give the illusion of productivity without achieving real outcomes; and 'taskmasters', who create unnecessary work for others. Crucially, Graeber suggests that even roles initially intended to fulfil important tasks can, through the way they are organised and deployed, become examples of 'bullshit' work. Nightingale's frustration with the unrequested influx of nurses, potentially valued more for the political optics they provided than for their actual contribution to patient care, offers an early historical illustration of this phenomenon. Crucially however, Graeber's theory suggests that whilst jobs often seek to do *genuinely* necessary or important things, the way they are conducted renders them bullshit and therefore within the taxonomy of jobs described here.

The significance of this theory in the contemporary nursing context has not gone unnoticed. In a provocatively titled article in the Nursing Inquiry '*on the bullshitisation of mental health nursing*'.[8] Mick McKeown provides his analysis of Graeberian bullshit in modern nursing. Acknowledging the likely initial reaction of many to the idea of any form of nursing being pointless as offensive, McKeown clearly states the inevitably disastrous consequences of eliminating these roles entirely; instead making a compelling argument that much of modern nursing work is, indeed, superfluous. His arguments principally consider the issues of record keeping becoming a *'bullshit proportion of the totality of nursing work'* in addition to the dissonance between the ideal of mental health nursing being a compassionate endeavour, and the reality that it is increasingly seen as coercive and restrictive. He estimates that around 50% of mental health nursing now comprises box-ticking and goonery. Nightingale certainly felt there was bullshit in the hospitals of the Crimea, describing the work of nurses in the hospital at Koulali as '*scampering about the wards ineffectually*'.[9] Arguably, there remains much bureaucratic inefficiency in nursing which could potentially be avoided.

To use one contemporary example, the current infection control nursing workforce is subject to much potential bullshit.* This is certainly an issue which would have bothered Nightingale. A Centre for Workforce Intelligence review[10] of the UK infection control nurse workforce in 2015 reported wide variations in practice, with no uniformity in person specification, competency, substantial variability in team structures and service delivery models and reported that infection control nurses have various remits and responsibilities, it is unknown how many infection control nurses there are in the UK. This lack of structure and clarity arguably left the health services in a poor condition to deal with the challenges of the COVID-19 pandemic five years later. In one of my own national studies in 2024,[11] looking at perceptions of outbreak management it was indicated that many organisations fail to collect sufficient data on outbreaks, do not evaluate their interventions and have relatively unstructured approaches to dealing with them. An indicative quote from one survey respondent stated:

> There is no set process established currently that enables effective outbreak management, the processes and guidelines required are unclear and appear to be reactive rather than proactive. Outbreak management presently seems driven more by organisational pressures than patient safety.
>
> (Infection control nurse)

It seldom needs stating that infectious disease requires careful consideration to prevent transmission and save lives. This was an issue central to Nightingale's philosophy of nursing and motivated her extensive efforts for sanitary reform. The efficacy of our current approaches to achieving this aim however, in addition to our broader nursing goals require careful reflection by modern nurses. Nightingale would likely be dissatisfied with the inconsistency, and at times, entirely valueless activities undertaken by nurses. This may be compounded in the contemporary context, where policymakers often use authoritative language such as 'must', 'should', 'will', and 'compliance' within policies, creating what has been described in contemporary research as a *fractured relationship between those who produce policies and the healthcare workers who need to comply with them*.[12] This distance may inadvertently generate further box-ticking activities, aiming to achieve a genuinely noble aim, but instead generating inefficiency, frustration, and distraction from a focus

---

* This is not to pick on a particular area of nursing, it just happens to be one which I am familiar with. As McKeown demonstrates, other areas of nurses are certainly not immune from bullshit.

on whether the practices being promoted genuinely work.[†] Ultimately, the clinical outcomes are the only indicator of the quality of nursing work and a reflection of the true value of the systems they work in. As Nightingale argued during her time tirelessly campaigning for improved conditions in India:

> We do not care for the people of India. This is a heavy indictment, but how else account for the facts about to be given?...Between five and six million have perished then in this Madras famine. These are figures, paper and print to us. How can we realise what the misery is of every one of those figures: a living soul, slowly starving to death?[13]

Systematic changes in modern nursing

By reflecting on current care processes and identifying systemic inefficiencies, nurses may continue to advocate for improved ways of providing nursing care. An example of this is the leadership of nurses on issues related to adoption novel technologies such as artificial intelligence or robotics into nursing practice. These technologies may offer entirely new services delivery models and opportunities to fundamentally change relationships between nurses and their patients. In work such as the Phillips-Ives review, led by nurses Dr Natasha Phillips (UK) and Dr Jeanette Ives Erickson (USA) which sought to identify what actions are needed to facilitate these system-wide changes.[‡] The report identified major educational gaps, made radical recommendations about the integration of new technologies into nursing practice including preparing students to operate in new care environments such as virtual wards (which were not, a remain, relatively rare within healthcare services). Nightingales' likely perspectives on these efforts to see care digitalised to facilitate reduced dependence on hospitals are evident in her writing:

> Hospitals are only an intermediate stage of civilization, never intended... to take in the whole sick population. May we hope that the day will come... when every poor sick person will have the opportunity of a share in a district sick nurse at home.[14]

Beyond the hospital walls, nurses today regularly engage in policy advocacy to address the social determinants of health, factors like poverty, education, and housing that affect patient outcomes. Just as Nightingale lobbied for reforms to improve environmental conditions, modern nurses are advocating for policies that tackle the root causes of poor health in communities. A key example of this is the Chief Nursing Officers for England's 2023 vision for nurses in

---

† Case in point – does infection control nurses spending time ensuring that staff on wards do not erect a Christmas tree *really* protect patients from infections?

‡ This review was witheld and later leaked to media outlets, echoing the controversy of Nightingale raising the alarm about conditions in military hospitals. See – 'Leaked NHSE review warns of 'severe' lack of nurses with digital skills' https://www.digital-health.net/2024/06/leaked-nhse-review-warns-of-severe-shortage-of-digital-nurses/

England which includes a new focus on planetary health as a focus of nurses. This represents an expansion even from that of Nightingale with her groundbreaking work on hospital design, to include issues such as climate change into the domain of nursing practice. Nightingale would no doubt approve of such changes, noting herself in her paper on 'Life or Death in India' that '*one must live in order to be a subject for sanitary considerations at all; and one must eat to live. If one is killed off by famine, one certainly need not fear fever or cholera*'.[15] Another key consideration of modern healthcare systems is the need to integrate an understanding of new digital environments, principally in the form of social media and how these interact with existing infrastructure and patients' health. Modern patients are subject to the influence of opaque algorithms and malign actors seeking to influence their behaviours.[16]

Modern nurses and their patients stand to benefit greatly from Nightingales focus on bureaucratic efficiency and attention to the harm caused by healthcare systems and more generally, the environments that patients exist within.

Key lessons for modern nurses to achieve the Nightingale Effect

- More nurses are not always the solution, effective role definition, competence and effective communication between components of the system are key.
- Nursing work is not free from 'bullshit', do not lose sight of the core purpose of nursing work and ensure that energy is not wasted on pointless activities which do not achieve the core nursing aim.
- Always address the root cause of inefficiencies, there is little point in focusing solely on compliance with policies if the clinical outcomes they seek to improve continue to get worse (or at least don't improve).
- Where inefficiencies are identified, they must be communicated effectively to those who may help affect change where needed.
- Consider how the patient environment may influence clinical outcomes, this may include consideration of new digital environments such as social media.

Some reflective questions to consider to help you on your way to improving systems of care:

1. What processes do you observe currently which would make no difference *to patients* if they were to cease?
2. What potential sources of harm are unrecognised by existing infrastructure?
3. If you had *complete* control over the system you work in, how would you design it?

References

1 Nightingale, F. (2022) *Notes on Hospitals*. BoD–Books on Demand.
2 *Army Sanitary Administration and Its Reform Under the Late Lord Herbert*. https://ia600202.us.archive.org/29/items/armysanitaryadmi00byunigh/armysanitaryadmi00byunigh.pdf
3 *Busting Bureaucracy: Empowering Frontline Staff by Reducing Excess Bureaucracy in the Health and Care System in England*. (2020, November 24). https://www.gov.uk/government/calls-for-evidence/reducing-bureaucracy-in-the-health-and-social-care-system-call-for-evidence/outcome/busting-bureaucracy-empowering-frontline-staff-by-reducing-excess-bureaucracy-in-the-health-and-care-system-in-england#conclusions
4 Nightingale, F. (1992). *Notes on Nursing*. Lippincott Williams & Wilkins.
5 Graeber, D. (2018). *Bullshit Jobs*. Simon & Schuster.
6 Nightingale, F. (1854). Signed letter, December 10 {f29v}, ff34–40v, pen, Goldie 50–52 [14:82–84]. https://bpb-ca-c1.wpmucdn.com/sites.uoguelph.ca/dist/3/30/files/2019/07/BL01GEN.pdf (From *Collected Works*, McDonald ed.)
7 Helmstadter, C. (2010). Navigating the political straits in the Crimean War. In Nelson, S., & Rafferty, A. M. (Eds.), *Notes on Nightingale: The Influence and Legacy of a Nursing Icon* (p. 34). ILR Press.
8 McKeown, M. (2023). On the bullshitisation of mental health nursing: A reluctant work rant. *Nursing Inquiry*, 31(1). Wiley. https://doi.org/10.1111/nin.12595
9 Bostridge, M. (2008). *Florence Nightingale: The Woman and Her Legend* (p. 243). Penguin.
10 *Centre for Workforce Intelligence Review of IPC Nursing Workforce* (2015). https://assets.publishing.service.gov.uk/media/5a7587b2e5274a545822c3b5/CfWI_Review_of_IPC_nurse_workforce.pdf
11 Wynn, M. (2024). Perceptions and digitalisation of outbreak management in UK health services: A cross-sectional survey. *Journal of Infection Prevention*, 25(4), 134–141. https://doi.org/10.1177/17571774241239221
12 Cole, M. A. (2015). A discourse analysis of hand hygiene policy in NHS Trusts. *Journal of Infection Prevention*, 16(4), 156–161. https://doi.org/10.1177/1757177415575412
13 Nightingale, F. (1878). *Collected Works – Excerpts on India*, 9:778 and 781. https://cwfn.uoguelph.ca/i-india/fn-excerpts-on-india/
14 Nightingale, F. (2004). Florence Nightingale on public health care. In McDonald, L. (Ed.), *Collected Works of Florence Nightingale* (p. 218). Wilfrid Laurier University Press.
15 Nightingale, F. (1873). *Life or Death in India*. Spottiswoode. https://en.wikisource.org/wiki/Life_or_Death_in_India
16 Garwood-Cross, L. (2025). The social media nurse. In Wynn, M. (Ed.), *Digital Nursing: Shaping Practice and Identity in the Age of Informatics* (pp. 72–86). Routledge.

3 Leadership through action, not hierarchy

Lead by Light, Not by Title

In mid-19th-century England, the societal norms and structures that governed women's lives were rigid and restrictive. Women, especially those of Florence Nightingale's class and stature, were typically confined to domestic roles, their ambitions stifled by societal expectations that prioritised marriage and motherhood over intellectual and professional pursuits. This period was marked by an overarching patriarchal authority that required women to seek permission for actions that today are considered basic rights. Florence Nightingale's aspirations to lead and innovate in nursing confronted these entrenched norms head-on. Despite her passion and vision for healthcare reform, her path was not straightforward or supported by the power structures of her time. In an era when women seldom held any formal authority in public spheres,[*] Nightingale had to navigate a labyrinth of social constraints. Her journey to the Crimean War, a pivotal moment in her career, reflected the extent of her challenges and limited personal autonomy: she required her parents' consent not only to travel but also to engage professionally in a war zone, an environment out of bounds for women of her era. Furthermore, her travels to and presence in Crimea had to be chaperoned, reflecting the prevailing belief that women needed protection and supervision, due to their perceived dependency and frailty.

Despite these barriers, Nightingale's leadership emerged not from a formal title or hierarchical power but through relentless action and commitment to improving healthcare. Her situation vividly illustrates that leadership can manifest through actions that challenge and eventually reshape existing structures, rather than through traditional authoritative roles. Nightingale didn't wait for military leaders to organise the hospital she arrived at in Scutari, or to improve conditions. She and her nurses began cleaning the hospital

---

[*] Women in Britain did not gain the right to vote until eight years after Florence Nightingale's death. Initially, only women over 30 with property qualifications could vote, with equal voting rights to men granted by the Equal Franchise Act of 1928.

DOI: 10.4324/9781003646259-4

Table 3.1 British Army Leadership Code (2016): Seven leadership behaviours[2]

1   Lead by example
2   Encourage thinking
3   Apply reward and discipline
4   Demand high performance
5   Encourage confidence in the team
6   Recognise individual strengths and weaknesses
7   Strive for team goals

themselves, scrubbing floors, changing bed linens, and reorganising the wards to ensure that soldiers had space and ventilation. She also implemented strict hygiene protocols, which drastically reduced infection rates. Nightingale's leadership was driven by a sense of *personal* responsibility to her patients. She embodied the principle that leadership in nursing is about seeing a problem, owning it, and taking decisive action to fix it. As she said in a lecture to her nurses in 1872:

> What are the qualities which give us authority, which enable us to exercise some charge or control over other with "authority"? It is not the charge or position itself, for we often see persons in a position of authority, who have no authority at all; and on the other hand, we sometimes see persons in the very humblest position who exercise a great influence or authority on all around them. The very first element for having control over others is, of course, to have control over oneself. If I cannot take charge or myself, I cannot take charge of others.[1]

> Nightingale – Lecture to her nurses 1872

This quote reflects one of the hallmarks of Nightingale's leadership was her ability to inspire others by leading through action. While many doctors and military officials initially resisted her reforms, Nightingale's tireless work ethic, dedication, and careful focus on negotiation gradually won them over. Her nightly rounds through the wards, where she checked on soldiers by the light of a small lamp, earned her the nickname '*The Lady with the Lamp*'. More than just a symbol of compassion, these rounds were an expression of her leadership philosophy: she was willing to do the hard, hands-on work herself, demonstrating personally what needed to be done. Crucially, as Nightingale observes, if one cannot take charge of themselves, it is not reasonable to expect others to take even greater charge than their leader. This very ethos remains a focus of the British Army's Leadership doctrine (see Table 3.1). The importance of role modelling is sadly often forgotten, particularly by those with formal authority, who may misunderstand their position as a right to automatic respect and effective followership.

Rebel nurse leadership: Making an impact without a title

Although women's rights and access to formal professions have improved significantly in many countries, nurses continue to face leadership challenges today. One of the most enduring of these is the fact that, despite their critical roles in healthcare delivery, most nurses do not occupy formal positions of authority within organisational hierarchies. Nightingale's example remains particularly powerful in this context: she demonstrated that leadership in nursing does not depend on titles or formal power, but on the ability to take decisive action, model the standards expected of others, and earn influence through self-discipline and visible commitment. In a profession where formal authority may not always be granted, the ability to lead through action and personal example remains central to effective nursing leadership.

This continuing need for nurses to exercise leadership without relying on formal authority has been recognised in contemporary scholarship. Building on examples like Nightingale's, modern researchers have developed the concept of 'rebel nurse leadership'.[3] Rebel nurse leaders are characterised by their unconventional and non-conformist behaviours, challenging established norms, practices, and strategies. They leverage social networks both within and beyond their organisations to access evidence-based knowledge, share information, and rally others in pursuit of better outcomes for patients and healthcare systems.[3] Rather than accepting organisational limitations, rebel nurse leaders find creative ways to lead and drive change from positions outside traditional hierarchies.

Nightingale was undoubtedly a 'rebel' nurse leader. The characteristics of these leaders and their positive and negative impacts were described by Eline de Kok and colleagues.[3] Crucially, it is possible to deviate negatively. Deviation from normal standards and approaches to practice may risk reputation, damage relationships and create unsustainable solutions. Four key competencies of effective rebel nurse leaders are suggested by de Kok et al., including:

1 Ability to communicate, sharing key information which challenges the status quo (this is addressed in more depth in Chapter 5).
2 An ability to work collaboratively with other professionals and people in positions of formal authority both within and outside of their organisations (this is addressed in more depth in Chapter 6).
3 The ability to critically assess and reflect on working practices and issues within processes.
4 The creative ability to generate innovative ideas (this is addressed in more depth in Chapter 7).

Effective rebel nurse leadership necessarily entails conflict, which nurses are, understandably, often unwilling to engage in.[4] This conflict is typically necessary to raise consciousness of potentially unworkable practices which nurses engage in to compensate for systemic issues within health services. In Nightingales context, the conditions at the hospital in Scutari entirely reflect this tension, whereby the medical and military establishment at the time wanted to maintain a sense of competence in their system of care. Contrasting strongly with Nightingale's observations of the conditions. In raising awareness of the conditions via meticulous data collection, shared with the relevant authorities, she was able to effect lasting change in approaches to managing care for soldiers.

Over the years since Nightingale's death, many theories of leadership have been described and variously come in and out of fashion.[5] Some nurse leaders may recall being asked to identify their 'leadership style', for example, 'transactional'[†] or 'transformational'.[‡] Crucially, nurses should avoid considering themselves to be restricted to one 'style'. Nightingale understood this, she may have exerted transactional leadership in maintaining discipline on her wards when dismissing drunken nurses,[§] whilst adopting a more transformational approach towards the systems she worked within. To use a medical analogy, a *diagnosis* of the *leadership situation* is needed to affect the most impactful change. Nightingales approach in this regard arguably reflects what has come to be referred to as 'meta-leadership', characterised by leadership which intentionally connects the work of different organisations and organisational units, thinking beyond one's immediate scope of authority and typical bureaucratic patterns of behaviour.[6] This often required what is referred to as 'leading down' (to subordinates), 'leading up' (to superiors), 'leading across' to peers and 'leading beyond' (to organisations outside of the leaders own).[7]

Nightingale's leadership transcended conventional boundaries, exemplifying the essence of meta-leadership through her mastery of self-discipline, strategic navigation of complex systems, and ability to build alliances across diverse organisational structures. Her seminal contributions in the Crimea, her reforms in India, and her foundational role in global nurse education were not isolated acts, but part of a cohesive leadership strategy that redefined healthcare and nursing. By dynamically integrating different leadership approaches based on contextual needs, Nightingale demonstrated a profound understanding of the complex interplay required to achieve systemic change, connecting disparate individuals and organisations towards unified, transformative goals.

---

† Focuses on supervision, organisation, and performance. Transactional leadership is responsive, and its effectiveness is based on a system of rewards and punishments.

‡ Inspires and motivates followers to innovate and create change. Transformational leadership enhances the motivation, morale, and performance of followers through a variety of mechanisms.

§ An alarmingly common feature of nursing at the time.

Key lessons for modern nurses to achieve the Nightingale Effect

- Leadership in nursing is about taking initiative and being proactive in solving problems. Lead by stepping forward to address issues directly, regardless of whether you have a formal authority position.
- Embrace a deep sense of personal responsibility for patient care and outcomes.
- Having control over oneself is essential to leading others effectively.
- Leadership involves critical thinking and questioning norms.
- Effective rebel leadership involves working collaboratively and communicating effectively with both peers and those in positions of formal authority. Sharing knowledge and engaging others are crucial for driving improvements and innovations in patient care.
- Demonstrate the behaviours you wish to see in others.
- Conflict is often inevitable to lead health systems towards sustainable change, anticipate this, and be prepared to demonstrate moral courage and persistence.
- Diagnosing the leadership situation is necessary to ensure approaches to leadership reflect the nuances of the socio-cultural context within which it is required.
- Aspire to be a meta-leader, consider how you may exert influence up, down, across, and beyond.

Reflective questions to consider to help you to lead by light:

1 What behaviours do I currently exhibit which I would not like to see in those leading me?
2 Who do I look up to as a leader, why?
3 What issues in nursing do I want people to take me more seriously on, and how might I make this happen?

References

1 Nightingale, F. (1915) *Nightingale to Her Nurses.* (p.12) Macmillan and Co.
2 *Army Leadership Code* (2016). https://www.army.mod.uk/support-and-training/our-schools-and-colleges/centre-for-army-leadership/leadership-resources/army-leadership-code/
3 de Kok, E., Weggelaar-Jansen, A. M., Schoonhoven, L., & Lalleman, P. (2021). A scoping review of rebel nurse leadership: Descriptions, competences and stimulating/hindering factors. *Journal of Clinical Nursing*, 30, 2563–2583. https://doi.org/10.1111/jocn.15765

4   de Kok, E., Schoonhoven, L., Lalleman, P., & Weggelaar, A. M. (2023). Understanding rebel nurse leadership-as-practice: Challenging and changing the status quo in hospitals. *Nursing Inquiry*, 30, e12577. https://doi.org/10.1111/nin.12577
5   Benmira, S., & Agboola, M. (2021). Evolution of leadership theory. *BMJ Leader*, 5(1), 3–5. https://doi.org/10.1136/leader-2020-000296
6   Marcus, L. J., Dorn, B. C., & Henderson, J. M. (2006). Meta-leadership and national emergency preparedness: A model to build government connectivity. *Biosecurity and Bioterrorism: Biodefense Strategy, Practice, and Science*, 4(2), 128–134. Mary Ann Liebert Inc. https://doi.org/10.1089/bsp.2006.4.128
7   McNulty, E., Marcus, L., Grimes, J., Henderson, J., & Serino, R. (2021, November 29). The meta-leadership model for crisis leadership. *Oxford Research Encyclopedia of Politics*. Retrieved 12 Mar. 2025, from https://oxfordre.com/politics/view/10.1093/acrefore/9780190228637.001.0001/acrefore-9780190228637-e-2032

4 Proactive detection and vigilance in care

See the Shadows before They Fall

> *Nightingale recognised that prevention was not just better than cure, it is both more efficient and humane.*
>
> It is much cheaper to promote health than to maintain people in sickness[1]
>
> (Florence Nightingale 1894)

Florence Nightingale is often remembered for her compassion and her tireless dedication to patient care, but one of her most valuable, and perhaps overlooked skills was her ability to observe. Nightingale understood that the key to improving patient outcomes wasn't just in dramatic medical interventions but in noticing the subtle, often small changes that could signal larger, life-threatening issues. This attention to detail continues to be a crucial skill for modern nurses today. Mastering the art of observation can mean the difference between early intervention and life-threatening escalation, and it is at the core of what makes a great nurse. In her own words:

The most important practical lesson that can be given to nurses is to teach them to observe-how to observe- what symptoms indicate improvement what the reverse- which are of importance-which are of none- which are the evidence of neglect- and what kind of neglect. If you cannot get into the habit of observation one way or another, you had better give up being a nurse. In dwelling upon the vital importance of sound observation, it must never be lost sight of what observation is for. It is not for the sake of piling up miscellaneous information or curious facts, but for the sake of saving life and increasing health and comfort[2]

DOI: 10.4324/9781003646259-5

The importance of vigilance in modern nursing

Observation remains one of the most important skills for modern nurses, particularly in clinical settings where the stakes are high. Nurses are often the first line of defence in identifying subtle changes in a patient's condition, which can signal the onset of a serious complication. Research consistently shows that early detection of subtle signs, such as minor changes in respiratory rate, skin colour, or mental status, can dramatically improve patient outcomes. For example, a slight increase in a patient's respiratory rate might seem insignificant on its own, but it can be an early sign of sepsis, a life-threatening condition if not caught and treated quickly. Nurses who are vigilant and notice these changes can initiate early interventions that save lives.

Technology as an aid, not a replacement for observation

While modern healthcare has benefited immensely from advancements in technology, including electronic health records, diagnostic tools, and monitoring systems, these tools should never replace the human element of observation. For example, nurses who rely solely on machines to monitor vital signs may miss important cues that technology can't pick up,* such as a patient's facial expression of discomfort or a subtle change in their voice that might indicate pain or anxiety. Without this crucial human judgement, much digital data collection in healthcare will amount to little more than '*piling up miscellaneous information or curious facts*' as Nightingale put it. There remains evidence that this Nightingalean wisdom still holds true today. In an extensive review of the literature of nurses' uses of Early Warning Scores (EWS), which are quantitative measures of key observations to identify patient deterioration, it was reported that nurses rely heavily on the scores themselves rather than utilising fully the clinical judgement of the nurse.[3] Potentially leading to late identification of deteriorating patients.

Florence Nightingale understood the importance of presence when observing patients closely. During her nightly rounds in the hospital, she would, famously, walk the wards with her lamp. This hands-on, vigilant approach allowed her to develop a deeper understanding of each patient's condition, creating a bond of trust with the soldiers, who knew she was paying close attention to their well-being. Today, nurses who master the balance between technology and hands-on observation are better equipped to provide comprehensive care. Despite advances in technological capability, the importance

---

* At least not for now, even as technology advanced, ensuring that the interpretation of data outputs from digital tools will likely always require a level of effective (i.e. not ritualised and unengaged) human oversight.

Table 4.1 Manifesting presence in the context of an online chat-based consultation

High presence	Mixed presence	Low presence
Nurse: "Hello Sarah, it's good to meet you. I see from your notes you've had some breathlessness lately, could you tell me more about when it started? Take your time. I'm here to help. Also, just checking, are you comfortable using this chat system, or would you prefer a quick call if it's easier?"	**Nurse:** "Hi Sarah. I see you've reported breathlessness; can you tell me how long you've been experiencing it? Please include any other symptoms. Thanks".	**Nurse:** "Hi. Describe symptoms. How long? Severity? Any medications?"
Explanation:	**Explanation:**	**Explanation:**
• The nurse personalises the greeting, refers specifically to the patient's problem, invites narrative (allowing trust to build), and shows flexibility with the medium. • **Manifestation of presence:** Active engagement, warmth, and adaptation to patient needs despite the digital barrier. • **Implications for preventative care:** Early trust and openness help uncover crucial symptoms or risks that the patient might otherwise omit, allowing proactive management.	• The nurse acknowledges the patient by name and refers specifically to the issue, showing *some* personalisation and attentiveness. However, the tone remains brisk and transactional, lacking emotional warmth or reassurance, and without checking on the patient's comfort with the communication method. • Manifestation of presence: Partial engagement. The patient may feel somewhat recognised but still sense a functional, task-focused interaction rather than genuine human concern. • Implications for preventative care: Some useful information may still be collected, but opportunities to uncover deeper issues (like anxiety about symptoms, hidden comorbidities, or early deterioration signs) could easily be missed. Trust-building is weaker than it could be, making follow-up or adherence to advice less reliable.	• The nurse's communication is curt, formulaic, and transactional, lacking empathy or human warmth. • **Manifestation of presence:** Minimal engagement; the patient feels like a data point rather than a person. • **Implications for preventative care:** Patients may give brief, incomplete answers, feel dismissed, and important warning signs (e.g., emotional distress, nuanced symptoms) could be missed, increasing the risk of preventable deterioration.

of presence has not diminished. Oil lamps and nightly rounds have been replaced by tools such as telemonitoring and teleconsultation technologies. Yet the need for nurses to be meaningfully 'present' remains vital. Contemporary nurse theorists, such as David Barrett, have explored how presence can be achieved within a technological context. Barrett identifies four key types of presence in digitally mediated care:[4]

1 Operational presence – Managing essential administrative functions, such as organising patient flow through teleconsultation clinics, setting up equipment, and troubleshooting telecoms systems.
2 Clinical presence – Competently performing clinical tasks such as history-taking, visual examination, providing advice, and prescribing care.
3 Therapeutic presence – Offering emotional support, providing reassurance, and recognising and responding to non-verbal cues.
4 Social presence – Engaging in informal conversation unrelated to the clinical purpose of the consultation. This can be enhanced by minimising the perceived distance created by technology, helping patients feel as if the nurse is truly 'in the room' with them.

Mastering these dimensions of presence allows modern nurses to maintain the compassionate, attentive ethos Nightingale exemplified, even when working through digital platforms. In telecommunications, presence refers not only to being available but to the sense of attentiveness and engagement that can be conveyed even through minimal or brief exchanges, something especially significant in digital contexts where communication is often decontextualised and stripped of non-verbal cues. Examples of high vs. low presence as mediated purely through an online chat-based consultation can be seen in Table 4.1.

There has been a proliferation of research focusing on the potential of machine learning and artificial intelligence to enhance patient monitoring in healthcare. While these technologies offer considerable benefits, it is important to recognise that the ritualised collection of patient data, often disconnected from genuine clinical insight, is not new. Florence Nightingale herself criticised such practices in her time. I have previously argued that as healthcare becomes increasingly digitalised, we must remain vigilant about the purpose of the data we collect and analyse and avoid simply transferring poor observational habits onto automated systems.[5] Although we tend to associate data with digital technologies today, every interaction with a patient is inherently a data-rich event. Every gesture, facial expression, and choice of words offers valuable information that, if interpreted thoughtfully, deepens our understanding of the patient. If we fail to engage with these human signals, as Nightingale warned, we risk abandoning the very essence of nursing. The lamp has become a screen, but the light must still come from us.

The subtle signs of mental health and emotional well-being

In addition to spotting physical changes, nurses must also be adept at recognising subtle signs of emotional or psychological distress in their patients. Mental health is often intertwined with physical health, and a patient who is anxious, depressed, or fearful may not always express these emotions openly. Nurses who are skilled in observation can pick up on non-verbal cues, such as a patient avoiding eye contact, seeming withdrawn, or displaying unusual agitation, and take appropriate action to address these concerns. Arguably, Nightingale was ahead of her time in recognising the importance of emotional well-being in patient recovery. It was not until 1977 when George Engel first popularised the idea of looking beyond purely biomedical approaches to care with his proposal of the 'biopsychosocial model'.[6] Recognising the importance of social and psychological influences on illness and 'patienthood'. Nightingale wrote extensively about the need for hospitals to provide a healing environment, noting that *'apprehension, uncertainty, waiting, expectation, fear of surprise, do a patient more harm than any exertion'.*[7]

She understood that emotional distress could delay recovery, something which has been extensively validated with modern research studies, and she used her observational skills to ensure that patients were not just physically cared for but emotionally supported as well. This came in addition to concerns over their social welfare, she regularly argued for better living conditions for soldiers, arguing that many of their less-healthy activities may be remedied by access to adequate opportunities for leisure. Modern nurses continue to follow this principle, particularly in environments where patients may be vulnerable to anxiety and stress. By recognising and addressing patients' emotional needs, nurses can help reduce stress and anxiety, which has been shown to improve recovery rates and overall patient satisfaction.

Preventative healthcare – the buck stops with nature

During a time before germ-theory and doctors were still undecided on the value of handwashing, Nightingale championed preventative care. Her conviction emerged from a particular philosophy: medicine does not cure; it merely removes barriers to nature's inherent healing power. As she wrote:

> It is often thought that medicine is the curative process. It is no such thing; medicine is the surgery of functions, as surgery proper is that of limbs and organs. Neither can do anything but remove obstructions; neither can cure; nature alone cures. What nursing has to do in either case, is to put the patient in the best condition for nature to act upon him.[7]

This is a lesson which remains true today. Whilst medicine has undoubtedly changed dramatically since Nightingale's time, there remain many things, particularly in relation to the activities of nurses, which remain largely primarily the domain of natural forces. Perhaps, ironically, the most obvious being our ongoing struggles to control epidemic infectious diseases. For example, despite nearly two centuries having passed since the significance of hand hygiene was revealed by Ignaz Semmelweis, adherence to guidelines is typically low. One recent study reported overall compliance with hand hygiene policies to be around 17%[8] Crucially, the issue of human nature and human behavioural change are the limiting factors, not our knowledge of biomedicine itself. Another example is wound dressings. Despite the grand claims, and competent marketing efforts of contemporary wound dressing companies, it remains the case that wound dressings cannot *heal* wounds. At best, they may facilitate the creation of wound conditions which allow the body to heal effectively. Nightingale recognised the importance of this distinction. To take another example, pressure ulcers (or bed sores as Nightingale referred to them) have long been considered, even by Nightingale, as an indicator of the quality of nursing itself. However, more recently, and controversially, it has been suggested that it may in fact not be the case that poor nursing care is primarily the cause of these injuries, but instead a range of intrinsic pathophysiological factors.[9] Many of which lie outside of the control of nurses. In the UK, nurses spend considerable time completing paperwork, collecting data, and investigating the development of such wounds. On average the National Health Service in the UK typically pays out around £16.8 million per year in litigation for these wounds.[10] Preventative care in this context often rests on assumptions about the effectiveness of nursing interventions, assumptions that warrant careful scrutiny.[†]

Importantly, Nightingale also cautioned against the mechanical collection of information purely for ritualistic compliance. She recognised the necessity for critical clinical judgement, emphasising that healthcare should never lose sight of the natural boundaries limiting human intervention. As healthcare providers, particularly nurses, we must thoughtfully distinguish between what we genuinely control and what ultimately remains in nature's hands. Ensuring that resources and time is not wasted invested in false perceptions about this balance.

Contemporary challenges in preventative healthcare remain significant and would likely have drawn Nightingale's attention were she alive today. She would undoubtedly be interested in the escalating threat of antibiotic resistance, the complex interplay of globalisation and infectious disease spread, and

---

[†] Readers are strongly encouraged to review the quality of evidence reported in the most recent Cochrane reviews as to the efficacy of current interventions in this area (and others) and form their own opinions as to how much confidence we should have in them. These are available at https://www.cochrane.org/

the impacts of climate change on population health. Nightingale would also have recognised the challenges presented by healthcare inequalities, exacerbated by socioeconomic disparities and limited access to preventative care. Additionally, modern epidemics such as obesity, diabetes, and mental health, alongside emerging diseases and vaccine hesitancy, illustrate the critical need for robust preventative strategies that align closely with Nightingale's foundational philosophies of care and proactive intervention.

Key lessons for modern nurses to achieve the Nightingale Effect

- Prevention is better than cure.
- Understanding the balance between the power of nature and the power of health professionals to intervene in disease is key to effective care and the avoidance of unhelpful ritual.
- Always ensure to apply proper judgement to assessment information, data can't interpret itself.
- Avoid collecting information which doesn't contribute towards improving patients' health.
- Despite the increasing digitalisation of nursing practice, maintaining an effective sense of presence remains both achievable and essential for gathering the information needed to prevent unnecessary patient deterioration.
- Holism is the key to effective patient care, always consider the whole patient and not just the disease.

Reflective questions to consider to help you to spot the subtle:

1 How do I account for changes in patient's conditions which machines and checklists can't account for?
2 How can I better understand the ongoing experiences of my patients whilst they are under my care?
3 How much of the data which my service collects are used usefully to improve patient care?

References

1 Nightingale, F. (1894). *Health and Local Government: Introduction to Report of the Bucks Sanitary Conference October 1894* (pp. i–ii). Poulton.
2 Karimi, H., & Masoudi Alavi, N. (2015). Florence Nightingale: The mother of nursing. *Nursing and Midwifery Studies*, 4(2), e29475. https://doi.org/10.17795/nmsjournal29475

3 Wood, C., Chaboyer, W., & Carr, P. (2019). How do nurses use early warning scoring systems to detect and act on patient deterioration to ensure patient safety? A scoping review. *International Journal of Nursing Studies*, 94, 166–178. Elsevier BV. https://doi.org/10.1016/j.ijnurstu.2019.03.012

4 Barrett, D. (2017). Rethinking presence: A grounded theory of nurses and teleconsultation. *Journal of Clinical Nursing*, 26, 3088–3098. https://doi.org/10.1111/jocn.13656

5 Wynn, M., Silva, T. H. R. D., & Pearson-Jenkins, J. (2025). Introduction to digital nursing and nursing theory. In *Digital Nursing* (pp. 1–26). Routledge. https://doi.org/10.4324/9781032714547-1

6 Engel, G. L. (1977). The need for a new medical model: A challenge for biomedicine. *Science*, 196(4286), 129–136.

7 Nightingale, F. (1992). *Notes on Nursing*. Lippincott Williams & Wilkins.

8 Haenen, A., de Greeff, S., Voss, A., et al. (2022). Hand hygiene compliance and its drivers in long-term care facilities: Observations and a survey. *Antimicrobial Resistance & Infection Control*, 11, 50. https://doi.org/10.1186/s13756-022-01088-w

9 Berlowitz, D. R., & Levine, J. M. (2025). The evolving case for skin failure—Beyond pressure injury. *JAMA Internal Medicine*. Published online January 13, 2025. https://doi.org/10.1001/jamainternmed.2024.7461

10 NHS Resolution. (2024). Response to FOI request in relation to litigation resulting from pressure injuries in the NHS. https://resolution.nhs.uk/wp-content/uploads/2024/12/FOI_6883_Pressure-Sores.pdf

5 Lifelong learning and evidence-based practice

Cultivate Knowledge as Your Greatest Tool

Florence Nightingale's legacy as the founder of modern nursing was not just rooted in her compassion or leadership but in her commitment to learning and evidence-based practice. This passion for learning extended far beyond the boundaries of clinical subjects. She took an interest in languages, mathematics, politics (particularly women's-rights), and philosophy. Notably, she had a close relationship with John Stuart Mill, a key proponent of utilitarian ethics, who offered Nightingale feedback on her philosophical writings. Her interest in learning and particularly her interest in philosophy likely provided her with significant advantages in the process of creative problem-solving. This would have especially been the case among her female peers, who at the time typically did not enjoy the privilege of a robust education, which Nightingale had received from her father.

In an era when healthcare was largely driven by tradition, intuition, and anecdotal evidence, Nightingale was an early adopter of a more scientific approach.* She meticulously collected and analysed data to inform her decisions, using evidence to advocate for systemic reforms that saved countless lives. For modern nurses, her example serves as a reminder that greatness in nursing is inextricably tied to continuous learning and the application of evidence-based practices.

Nightingale's use of evidence: a revolution in nursing

Florence Nightingale's work during the Crimean War is perhaps the most well-known example of her dedication to evidence-based practice. Rather than relying on the prevailing medical wisdom of the time, which often overlooked environmental factors in patient care, Nightingale applied a data-driven approach. She meticulously tracked mortality rates, infection

---

* The concept of 'evidence-based medicine' was not popularised until Gordan Guyatt coined the term in a 1991 editorial. See. Guyatt, G. H. (1991). Evidence-based medicine. *ACP Journal Club*, *114* (2), A-16.

DOI: 10.4324/9781003646259-6

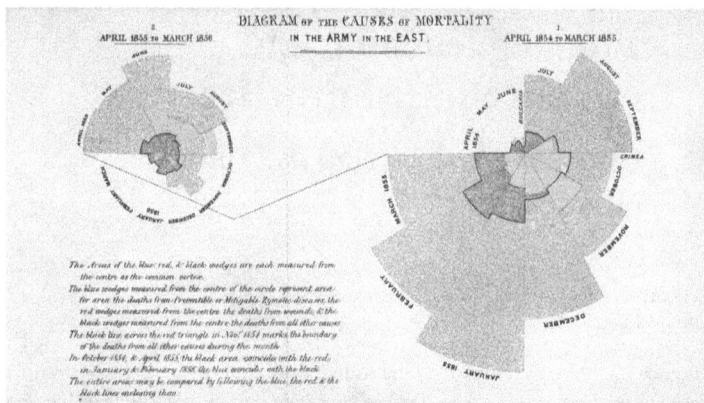

Figure 5.1 Diagram of the causes of mortality in the army in the East (1858) by Florence Nightingale

rates, and the overall health of the soldiers in her care. Her famous 'coxcomb' diagrams were a visual representation of the data she collected, showing how improvements in sanitation and hospital conditions could dramatically reduce death rates (see Figure 5.1). Through these diagrams, Nightingale was able to prove to British officials that the unsanitary conditions of the hospitals were associated with the high mortality rates. Her advocacy, supported by hard evidence, led to sweeping reforms in military hospitals, drastically reducing the death rate. She actively promoted the avoidance of fallacious reasoning when it came to understanding clinical phenomena, as she warned in her Notes on Nursing:

> Almost all superstitions are owing to bad observation, to the post hoc, ergo propter hoc; and bad observers are almost all superstitious. Farmers used to attribute disease among cattle to witchcraft; weddings have been attributed to seeing one magpie, deaths to seeing three; and I have heard the most highly educated now-a-days draw consequences for the sick closely resembling these[1]

Nightingale's example highlights the enduring reality that those who combine practical knowledge with robust evidence gain the intellectual authority needed to lead real change. Too often nurses are aware of problems within healthcare systems, but this knowledge remains confined to frustrated discussions between nurses. As the adage goes *'no data, no problem'*. Data are not just counts of arbitrary occurrences or for simply generating interesting statistical insights *'miscellaneous information or curious facts'*. They are a tool which can be wielded to demonstrate to others the seriousness and the necessity of change within healthcare systems. Nurses in positions of formal authority may be frustrated by being *in authority* without being *authoritative*, should insufficient time been spent developing a robust theoretical knowledge, rhetorical skill, and mastery of key evidence with which to build compelling arguments to others.

Lifelong learning: beyond formal education

Florence Nightingale's commitment to learning extended far beyond her formal training. After the Crimean War, she continued to study and deepen her understanding of healthcare, focusing on areas such as public health, hospital design, and patient care. She wrote extensively on the importance of education for nurses and championed the idea that learning should be a lifelong pursuit. In a lecture to her nurses, Nightingale urged: 'Let us never consider ourselves finished nurses... we must be learning all of our lives'.[2]

This philosophy remains crucial for nurses today. Formal education provides a necessary foundation, but it is only the beginning. Nurses must commit to ongoing professional development through continuing education courses, conference participation, and keeping abreast of the latest research. In the digital age, access to online learning resources, research databases, and professional networks has made lifelong learning more accessible than ever. Nurses who stay current with new findings and innovations are better equipped to deliver high-quality, evidence-based care, directly improving patient outcomes.

Perhaps most importantly, it is the attitude towards self-directed learning, the willingness to pursue knowledge beyond the boundaries of formal education, that shapes the greatest professional impact. It is worth remembering that Nightingale herself did not benefit from anything resembling the structured, professionally guided education available to modern nurses. Her achievements were fuelled by an enduring commitment to learning, a mindset that remains as vital today as it was in her time.

The role of technology in continuous learning

Nightingale's use of data and statistics to inform her practice was groundbreaking for her time, and modern nurses can build on this legacy by embracing the technological tools available today. The advent of electronic health records (EHRs), digital diagnostics, and real-time patient monitoring systems allows nurses to collect and analyse data more effectively than ever before. These tools not only help in delivering more personalised and precise care but also offer opportunities for learning and improvement. For example, nurses may use EHRs to track patient outcomes over time, analysing data to identify trends or patterns that might inform changes in care protocols. This real-time data can be used to make evidence-based decisions that improve patient care.

However, as technology continues to evolve, nurses must stay updated on how to use these tools effectively. Despite these opportunities, there is evidence that nurses rarely seek to learn from these potentially rich sources of information about their patients. In the UK, a recent investigation of the National Health Service reported that despite the opportunities presented by digital technologies, they have 'not radically reshaped services',[3] and that data from digital systems are largely untapped for research. These technologies are ripe for great nurses to develop new insights into patient care. Had Nightingale lived in the age of digital technologies, she would undoubtedly have pioneered their use for the deeper understanding they could provide into patient well-being. Virtual environments such as social media, for instance, now offer new territories where care can be delivered, health can be studied, and patient experiences can be better understood.

Yet Nightingale's enduring impact was not solely rooted in her mastery of data or practice innovation, it was equally in her ability to communicate her insights compellingly. She understood that even the most revolutionary ideas would achieve little unless they were effectively shared and advocated for. Although she did not explicitly outline writing and public speaking as pillars of her nursing philosophy, her prolific writings and public efforts made clear that these skills were critical for advancing both practice and policy.

Writing as a tool for change

Words alone are often little more than air. Unless you are already in a position of formal autocratic authority or simply defending ideas which have already been committed to written language, speaking alone is often of little consequence. Writing has always been a powerful tool to organise and develop complex thoughts, reflect on experiences, and influence a broader audience. For Nightingale, writing was not just about documentation; it was about creating a compelling narrative that could convince even the most resistant institutions to adopt necessary changes. Her book, *Notes on Nursing: What It Is and What It Is Not*,[†] was revolutionary not only because it addressed critical nursing practices, but also because it presented these ideas in a way that was accessible to a wider audience, from nurses to policymakers. In today's world, writing is even more critical. Nurses are not only prac-

---

† This book sold 15,000 copies in the first month alone, modern nursing scholars could only dream of such sales figures.

titioners of care but also advocates, educators, and innovators. Writing helps nurses articulate their experiences, share evidence-based practices, and advocate for systemic reforms. Whether through articles, research papers, policy proposals, or even social media posts, writing enables nurses to share their insights and innovations with a global audience, thus accelerating progress in healthcare. The ability to distil complex ideas into simple, compelling formats is a skill every nurse can benefit from in today's evidence-based healthcare environment.

Despite Nightingales obsession with writing, she was not always necessarily the most rhetorically capable. According to biographer Mark Bostridge '*Nightingale's epistolary world is one of black and white values with few intermediate greys*'.[4] This perhaps reflects the passion with which Nightingale addressed the issues she saw in the world. Despite this very human flaw, she was still able to effectively win the support of key people via her writing which allowed her to achieve what she did. The lesson in this for modern nurses is clear, first, even poorly made or over-dramatic arguments may be persuasive, and second, ideally have others review writing before sharing it to ensure it is as balanced as possible. The later was indeed something Nightingale sought. Her 'suggestions for thought', an extensive, and somewhat controversial, collection of reflections on theological issues remained unpublished during her lifetime. Perhaps due to the mixed feedback she had received by several pre-eminent academics at the time.

The power of public speaking

In addition to writing, public speaking has long been a way to inspire, inform, and lead. While Nightingale was more known for her writing, she was also involved in public advocacy through lectures. Public speaking allows nurses to share their ideas in a more dynamic and engaging format, reaching audiences that written materials might not. For modern nurses, public speaking is an invaluable skill that extends beyond the traditional confines of nursing. Public speaking platforms, whether at conferences, webinars, or health forums, allow nurses to engage directly with both colleagues and the broader community, advocating for improvements in patient care, policy changes, or addressing emerging healthcare challenges. Moreover, the digital era has expanded these opportunities. Virtual platforms allow for real-time engagement across global audiences. TED Talks, webinars, and podcasts are just a few examples of how nurses can use public speaking to spread their messages far beyond their immediate workplaces. Social media platforms such as X or LinkedIn also enable nurses to participate in live discussions and thought leadership in real-time.

Despite the well-established utility of public speaking and its necessity as a leader,‡ the ability of nurses to speak publicly is not always explicitly recognised in nursing curricula. In the UK, for example, the ability to speak publicly is not described within the Future Nurse Curriculum.[5] Nor is emphasis placed on the ability to create compelling arguments in written formats, with the only writing skills promoted focussing on clinical documentation or patient information. These omissions may reflect an inadvertent signal that these skills are considered of lesser importance, potentially denying opportunities for new nurses to develop Nightingalean writing and speaking abilities. Complicating this further, fear of public speaking, also known as glossophobia, is not uncommon. This is also more common in women than men, in fact, it has been shown to be the strongest predictor of public speaking anxiety.[6] These challenges strongly indicate the need for special focus on this skill among nurses. Addressing glossophobia explicitly within nurse education through targeted interventions, such as actively creating opportunities to practice this skill, could reduce anxiety, fostering greater self-assurance and professional presence. In doing so, nursing education would not only address existing skill deficits but actively prepare nurses to engage meaningfully in shaping the future healthcare landscape, embodying Nightingale's legacy of advocacy and persuasive communication.

The necessity of knowledge sharing in modern nursing

For greatness in nursing to be achieved, new knowledge and ideas must not remain siloed or confined to individual institutions. Nurses must take ownership of disseminating their knowledge through both formal and informal channels. The interconnectedness of modern healthcare systems means that advancements in one area, when shared effectively, can influence practices worldwide. However, for knowledge sharing to be effective, nurses must refine their communication skills. It's not enough to have a great idea; it must be clearly communicated. Writing helps nurses clarify their ideas, develop evidence-based arguments, and propose actionable solutions. Public speaking, on the other hand, brings those ideas to life and allows for engagement with the audience, encouraging dialogue, collaboration, and feedback.

---

‡ Throughout my military career, from leadership courses as a non-commissioned officer through to my later training as a commissioned officer, the ability to communicate effectively through public speaking was regarded as an essential prerequisite for any position of formal authority. Leadership without effective verbal skills is like assessing a patient without speaking to them: essential information is lost, trust is weakened, and outcomes are compromised.

Key lessons for modern nurses to achieve the Nightingale Effect

- Influence requires knowledge, developing and continuously updating evidence-based knowledge gives your voice credibility and persuasive power.
- Intellectual authority is earned not by completing formal education, but by sustaining a lifelong, proactive commitment to learning, critical thinking, and professional growth.
- Communication is vital, strong writing and speaking skills transform knowledge into a compelling catalyst for change.
- Confront fears proactively, public speaking anxiety (glossophobia) is common, especially among women; actively practising this skill can significantly reduce anxiety and boost confidence.
- Leverage technology, modern digital health records and analytics represent an untapped resource, rich with opportunities to discover new insights and improvements in patient care.
- Share to learn, true institutional advancement relies on actively sharing knowledge, not merely accumulating it individually.

Reflective questions to consider to help you cultivate knowledge as a tool

1 How regularly do I engage with current nursing research or evidence-based practice developments, and how do I integrate this new knowledge into my practice?
2 What actions have I taken to improve my writing and public speaking skills?
3 If presented with evidence that could significantly improve patient outcomes, how confident do I feel in my ability to persuade colleagues or managers to adopt new practices? What could help build that confidence?

References

1 Nightingale, F. (1992). *Notes on Nursing.* Lippincott Williams & Wilkins.
2 Nightingale, F. (1915). *Nightingale to Her Nurses.* Macmillan and Co.
3 Darzi, A. (2024). *Independent Investigation of the National Health Service in England.* https://assets.publishing.service.gov.uk/media/66f42ae630536cb92748271f/Lord-Darzi-Independent-Investigation-of-the-National-Health-Service-in-England-Updated-25-September.pdf
4 Bostridge, M. (2008). *Florence Nightingale: The Woman and Her Legend* (p. 8). Penguin.
5 Nursing and Midwifery Council (2018). *Future Nurse: Standards of Proficiency for Registered Nurses.* https://www.nmc.org.uk/globalassets/sitedocuments/education-standards/future-nurse-proficiencies.pdf
6 Lintner, T., & Belovecová, B. (2024). Demographic predictors of public speaking anxiety among university students. *Current Psychology,* 43, 25215–25223. https://doi.org/10.1007/s12144-024-06216-w

6 Collaboration across disciplines

Weave connections, create unbreakable bonds

> *Nightingale knew that hospitals were more than buildings, they are living systems, reliant on collaboration. Her vision reminds us that healthcare progress depends on unity, not isolation.*
>
> Every hospital is an 'Association' in itself...to make progress possible, we must make this interdependence a source of good: not a means of standing still[1]
>
> Nightingale – Lecture to her nurses 1888

One of Nightingales most effective and strategic qualities was her ability to build alliances across disciplines. She understood that nursing, medicine, and healthcare policy should not operate in silos and that true progress requires collaboration. She not only revolutionised nursing by elevating its professional standards, but also worked closely with others to ensure her healthcare reforms were grounded in science and had lasting impact. In the same way, nurses today must foster collaborative relationships with their peers, interdisciplinary teams, and professional organisations to drive progress and improve patient care.

The power of networks

During the Crimean War, Nightingale quickly realised that improving sanitation and hospital care required not just nursing skills but collaboration with doctors, hospital administrators, and military officials. This ability to network was one of the key reasons she was able to introduce systemic reforms in hospital conditions and Nightingale's network was extensive.* Her most notable

---

* An interesting mapping of Nightingales network, created by researchers Altea Lorenzo-Arribas and Pilar Cacheiro can be seen at http://bit.ly/FNegonet See. Lorenzo-Arribas, A. and Cacheiro, P. (2020), Florence Nightingale's network: Women, power, and scientific collaboration. *Significance*, 17: 22–25.

DOI: 10.4324/9781003646259-7

collaborations were with John Sutherland and William Farr, both pioneering scientists. Farr helped Nightingale apply data to her observations, and together, they used statistics to highlight the preventable causes of death among soldiers. The data they collected demonstrated the link between poor sanitary conditions and high mortality rates, providing irrefutable evidence to policymakers and medical leaders. Recognition of the statistical capabilities Nightingale developed in this way were recognised in her lifetime via a fellowship of the Royal Statistical Society in 1858, making her the first women to achieve this accolade. In 1874 she was also made an honorary member of the American Statistical Association.

In addition to working with statisticians, Nightingale developed relationships with policymakers to ensure that the changes she implemented would be institutionalised. Her famous report on hospital conditions, based on data collected during the Crimean War, was presented to the British government and led to sweeping healthcare reforms. Her networks extended far beyond nursing and medicine; she cultivated relationships with influential figures such as Sidney Herbert, Secretary of State at War from 1852 to 1855) who championed her work and helped secure resources for reform.

Crucially, Nightingale recognised that while identifying and collecting data, and persuasive communication through written mediums, are important, they are not enough to create meaningful change. As she put it '*A report is not self-executive, and when the report is ended, the work begins*'.[2] This timeless wisdom highlights that working across professional boundaries is essential not only to properly diagnose and identify potential solutions to challenges, but also to ensure that these solutions are implemented through collaboration.

Modern collaborative nursing: the power of interdisciplinary teams

Nurses today are naturally positioned at the intersection of multiple disciplines. They work closely with doctors, pharmacists, social workers, and other healthcare professionals to provide holistic care to patients. Interdisciplinary collaboration is essential in modern healthcare because it leverages the expertise of each team member to improve patient outcomes. For example, in hospital settings, nurses often act as the primary communicators between patients and the broader healthcare team. Their role is to ensure that doctors, specialists, and allied health professionals are all on the same page regarding a patient's care plan. However, in a modern context, the necessity for nurses to work outside their immediate professional boundaries is more important than ever. This is due to three key changes in healthcare since Nightingale's time. First, from a clinical perspective, patients tend to live longer and therefore have more complex comorbidities including chronic diseases which typically require support from multiple professional groups. Second, advances in medical science have created far more diagnostic and therapeutic opportunities which may necessitate the involvement of multiple professions. Finally, advances in technology have created new actual, or potential solutions to address the growing complexity of healthcare.

These factors, taken together, illustrate how necessary effective collaboration is to address challenges in healthcare. In Nightingale's time, working outside of her professional boundaries may have involved statisticians, politicians, physicians, sociologists, and engineers to achieve her goals. Modern nurses have an entirely new selection of potential collaborators, including software engineers, data analysts, health economists, pharmaceutical industry leaders among many others. The complexity inherent in such collaborative work necessitates reflection on the boundaries of the nurse's knowledge and skill, to identify where the contributions of other groups may be needed. This is illustrated well within a contemporary nursing theory in the context of developing new nursing technologies developed by Kissa Bahari and colleagues, named 'Nursing Technologies Creativity as an Expression of Caring'.[3] This model can be seen in Figure 6.1.

As can be seen within the model, the nurse requires 'innovator characteristics' (more is covered in relation to innovation in nursing in Chapter 7) but critically, this does not require the skills to necessarily *create* the innovation independently. Bahari and colleagues describe these nurse innovator characteristics as:

1   Thinking outside the box
2   Positive emotional engagement
3   Team synergy

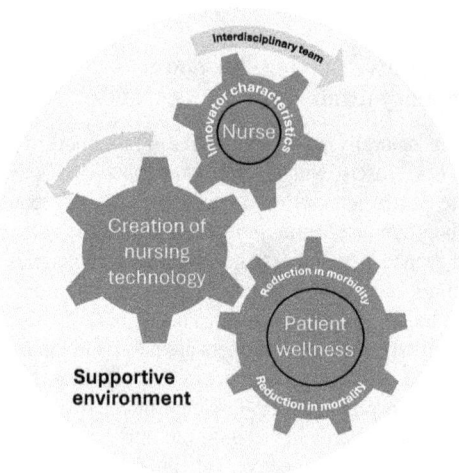

Figure 6.1 The theoretical model of technological creativity as caring in nursing (adapted from Bahari et al. 2021)

The ability to generate team synergy relies on an ability to communicate, loyalty, open-mindedness, cooperation, ability to coordinate teams, and manage interpersonal relationships. Arguably, these were the same skills required in Nightingale's time. Importantly, it is not necessary for nurses to have great technical skills themselves. Only an ability to recognise the nature of problems, coherently communicate these to those with the necessary skills to help solve them, and to bring these parts together to achieve the end goal. Namely, improved clinical outcomes; represented in the theory by the final cog indicating the impact of innovation on morbidity and mortality.

The role of professional networks and organisations

Beyond the bedside, nurses may also benefit from participating in professional organisations and building networks within the nursing community. Florence Nightingale understood the value of professional networks long before the nursing profession had formal structures in place. One of her lasting legacies was the founding of the Nightingale School of Nursing at St. Thomas' Hospital in London. By formalising nursing education, she created a network of trained nurses who could carry her vision forward. This was more than just a training school; it was a professional community that would continue to advocate for healthcare reforms and improve nursing standards globally. By the end of the 19th century, nurses trained at the Nightingale school were represented in hospitals across Europe, the Americas, Australasia, Asia and Africa. Several of whom she continued to correspond with to maintain her influence and understanding of nursing activities beyond her physical domain.

Today, professional organisations such as the American Nurses Association (ANA), the International Council of Nurses (ICN), and the Royal College of Nursing (RCN) play a critical role in supporting the professional development of nurses. These organisations provide opportunities for networking, continuing education, and advocacy, allowing nurses to stay informed about the latest research and policy changes. They also offer a platform for collective action, where nurses can advocate for better working conditions, patient safety standards, and healthcare reforms at local, national, and international levels. For example, during the COVID-19 pandemic, nursing organisations played a vital role in advocating for personal protective equipment (PPE), safe working conditions, and policy changes to protect both healthcare workers and patients. These organisations also facilitated the sharing of best practices and research on managing the virus, creating a collaborative network that spanned across borders. The ability to mobilise a global community of healthcare professionals in the face of a pandemic mirrors Nightingale's ability to leverage her networks for systemic change in healthcare.

Florence Nightingale's success in transforming healthcare wasn't solely due to her nursing expertise; it was her ability to build strong, collaborative networks that ensured her reforms had a lasting impact. Nurses today can learn from her example by fostering relationships with colleagues across disciplines, participating in professional organisations, and engaging in policy advocacy. By embracing collaboration, nurses not only enhance their own practice but also contribute to the advancement of the profession and the improvement of healthcare systems worldwide. Nightingale is sometimes referred to as a nurse *and a statistician*, this, I believe, is a false way to view her. She was a nurse, who utilised the statistics to further knowledge and practice within nursing. In this, it was her nursing identity, which was of most relevance, her interdisciplinary work with statisticians did not erode a nursing identity or add a new one, it merely made her nursing work *greater*.

Key lessons for modern nurses to achieve the Nightingale Effect

- Collaboration extends impact, nurses multiply their effectiveness when they engage and collaborate across disciplines.
- Effective collaboration requires nurses not necessarily to possess all technical skills, but the skill to bring diverse experts together to create solutions.
- Professional networks and nursing organisations empower nurses to influence healthcare on a broader scale, through education, advocacy, and collective action.
- Interdisciplinary collaboration should enrich nursing practice without diluting nursing identity.
- Nurses should confidently position their unique clinical insights as central to the collaborative process, reinforcing their professional role and expertise.

Reflective questions to consider to help you to cultivate knowledge as a tool

1. What complex problems do I regularly encounter in my practice that cannot be resolved by nursing expertise alone?
2. Who outside of nursing (e.g., technology experts, data analysts, pharmacists, engineers, policymakers) could I collaborate with to address these challenges effectively?
3. In what ways can I cultivate innovative thinking and team synergy within my clinical team or wider professional network to drive positive changes in patient care?

References

1 Nightingale, F. (1915). *Nightingale to Her Nurses* (p. 140). Macmillan and Co.
2 Nightingale, F. (1863). Letter to J. McNeil. In Vallée, G. (Ed.), *Florence Nightingale on Health in India* (p. 220). Wilfrid Laurier University Press, 2006.
3 Bahari, K., Talosig, A. T., & Pizarro, J. B. (2021). Nursing technologies creativity as an expression of caring: A grounded theory study. *Global Qualitative Nursing Research*, 8, 2333393621997397. https://doi.org/10.1177/2333393621997397

7 Innovating with lessons from history

Carve new visions from the stones of the past

>...what we need today is less of the icon and more of the iconoclast[1]
>
> Rafferty and Wall (2010) – Notes on Nightingale

Florence Nightingale didn't just create modern nursing; she transformed healthcare by challenging the status quo and introducing innovative practices that revolutionised patient care, hospital design, and public health. Her ability to think beyond the limitations of her time, using data, observation, and creativity, made a lasting impact on healthcare systems and established her as a pioneer of innovation in nursing. For nurses today, Nightingale's legacy is a powerful reminder that innovation is not just about technology or equipment but also about rethinking existing systems and processes to create lasting, meaningful change. One of Florence Nightingale's most famous innovations was her transformation of hospital design, best documented in her 'Notes on Hospitals' which became a guide to architects internationally.[*] She redesigned hospital spaces to optimise patient care and reduce infections, introducing what became known as the 'Nightingale Ward', a long, open room with large windows to allow natural light and fresh air, and beds spaced far apart to prevent the spread of infections. This design not only improved patient outcomes but also laid the foundation for modern hospital architecture, where patient safety and infection control are key considerations.

Of course, Nightingale was not the only nurse to innovate. In the decades since her death, many nurses have been associated with lasting innovations in

---

[*] Perhaps the most notable example was Nightingale's direct influence through her correspondence with Dr. John Shaw Billings. His design for what would become the internationally renowned Johns Hopkins Hospital was selected as the best of five submissions, but only after he had consulted directly with Nightingale on his plans.

See. Cope, Z. (1957). John Shaw Billings, Florence Nightingale and the Johns Hopkins Hospital. *Medical History*, 1(4), 367–368.

DOI: 10.4324/9781003646259-8

healthcare. Notable examples include Elise Sørensen, inventor of the colostomy bag in the 1950s; Anita Dorr, inventor of the 'crash cart' in the 1960s. In more recent times, we have witnessed the emergence of nurse founders of technology companies. With nurses converting their experience and insight into nursing problems into new technological solutions addressing issues from staffing to developing smartphone applications and hardware to support clinical activities. Undoubtedly the coming years will see an increasing number of nurses embrace artificial intelligence to address pressing issues in healthcare. An opportunity Nightingale would no doubt have embraced. The nature of innovation has changed somewhat since Nightingale's time. While her innovations in hospital design, patient care, and public health were revolutionary, they emerged within a context very different from today's healthcare landscape. Unlike contemporary nurse innovators, Nightingale operated in an era without structured support systems or opportunities for entrepreneurial endeavours. Innovation in her time often required navigating significant societal, institutional, and cultural barriers, with limited avenues for commercialisation or widespread implementation beyond direct advocacy and government influence.

In contrast, the contemporary environment for nursing innovation increasingly includes entrepreneurship as a viable and celebrated pathway. Nurses today can access structured mentorship programmes, startup incubators, and funding platforms specifically tailored for healthcare innovation. This entrepreneurial ecosystem has led to an exciting proliferation of nurse-led enterprises and startups, enabling the rapid translation of bedside insights into commercially viable products and technologies. Modern nurse innovators frequently blend clinical expertise with entrepreneurial acumen, actively contributing to transformative solutions such as telemedicine platforms, wearable health technology, digital record-keeping systems, and AI-driven decision-support tools.

The rise of entrepreneurialism provides nurses with a powerful new avenue to scale and disseminate innovations, extending their influence far beyond traditional healthcare settings. However, the fundamental ethos remains aligned with Nightingale's original vision: nurses are uniquely positioned to identify systemic challenges and creatively devise practical solutions. By embracing entrepreneurialism, nurses today carry forward Nightingale's legacy, demonstrating that innovation is fundamentally about challenging established norms, carving new visions from the stones of the past, and continually advancing healthcare practice through courageous creativity and determined advocacy. This link was reflected in a 2019 article by Johnson & Johnsons, a multinational pharmaceutical biotechnology and medical technologies corporation, who referred explicitly to contemporary nurse innovators as '*modern day Nightingales*'.[2] Given the changes in the innovation landscape however, further consideration of how nurses might innovate is warranted.

Modern nursing innovation: rethinking patient care in the age of the nurse entrepreneur

In the previous chapter, some of the characteristics of nurse innovators were described, specifically thinking outside of the box, positive emotional engagement the ability to create and lead teams. Although, this is not a complete picture. As in Nightingales time, an ability to communicate effectively via written and verbal methods remains essential. However, to generate lasting changes in practice at scale typically requires additional, complementary skills. Specifically, business acumen. Whether nurses intend to start their own business, or innovate to improve services they already work in, business literacy is a necessity. Ideally, innovations should achieve three aims, reduce costs, improve quality and improve access to healthcare. To achieve lasting innovation, many of the skills and attributes described in earlier chapters of this book are required. A basic outline of the process can be seen below:†

1 *Identify the Problem Clearly*
    Effective innovation begins by clearly defining a specific problem in clinical practice or patient care. Use direct observation and experience from your nursing practice to ensure you fully understand the issue.
2 *Gather Evidence and Insight*
    Collect evidence through reviews of literature, analysis of relevant data, and consultation with colleagues and patients. Understanding the historical context and previous attempts to solve similar issues will help you avoid repeating mistakes of the past and allow you to build upon proven concepts. Publicly available data may also provide further insights into the nature of the problem.
3 *Ideate and Conceptualise Solutions*
    Use creative thinking and brainstorming techniques, be bold, taking inspiration from historical nurse innovators like Nightingale. Explore diverse ideas, encourage yourself to think unconventionally. You will need to convince others that your solution is viable. This will require you to communicate its potential benefits effectively. This may involve managing the conflicting interests of parties who may wish to maintain the status quo. Nightingale experienced this prior to publication of her famous polar area diagrams which threatened to expose the inadequacy of existing

---

† There are many organisations dedicated to supporting nurses and other health professionals to successfully innovate. In the UK this includes the NHS Innovation service and regional health innovation networks. It is worth searching for relevant local organisations who may support this type of activity.

healthcare infrastructure. Making change often involves conflict. As discussed in Chapter 3, such conflict is often essential to lead meaningful change. At this stage, it is also important to consider intellectual property rights related to the potential solution. This is not always relevant, but failing to consider it could have catastrophic consequences for your innovation.

4 *Evaluate Feasibility and Impact*

Critically assess your ideas against practical considerations: Will they reduce costs, improve quality, and enhance access to healthcare? Evaluate your solution's feasibility, including clinical, economic, and organisational factors.

5 *Develop Business Literacy and Entrepreneurial Skills*

Acquire basic business knowledge, including project management, budgeting, funding strategies, and the essentials of scaling your idea. Even if you do not start your own business, understanding these skills is crucial to successful innovation. This will almost certainly require engagement with business experts and individuals who have successfully achieved lasting innovation previously. As discussed in the previous chapter, draw on the expertise and skill of others to support your work.

6 *Pilot and Iterate*

Test your innovation on a small scale, collect feedback, and refine your approach based on evidence and real-world experience. Be prepared to iterate multiple times to improve your concept.

7 *Scale and Sustain*

Once refined, plan for wider implementation, consider how the cost of your innovation (if any) will be accounted for over the long-term. Effective communication, leadership, and advocacy skills are essential to engage stakeholders and embed your innovation sustainably into practice.

Florence Nightingale's legacy reminds us that truly transformative change arises not only from bold ideas but from the relentless pursuit of practical solutions grounded in real-world needs. Today, the stones of the past, her pioneering reforms in design, hygiene, data use, and advocacy, remain foundational for nurses shaping the future. But the landscape has evolved. Innovation now demands fluency not only in clinical insight but also in the languages of business, entrepreneurship, and systems leadership. By combining the moral courage of historical nurse reformers with the strategic thinking and collaborative skills required in modern innovation ecosystems, nurses can continue to challenge the status quo. The enduring lesson is this: whether through redesigning hospitals or reshaping digital systems, innovation begins at the bedside, with the nurse who sees a problem, believes it can be solved, and dares to carve a new vision from the unyielding stone of established practice.

Key lessons for modern nurses to achieve the Nightingale Effect

- Define the problem, innovation begins with a precise understanding of a specific clinical issue or need.
- Gather data, review existing literature, and learn from past efforts to shape informed solutions.
- Embrace unconventional thinking to generate original ideas, take inspiration from historical nurse innovators.
- Critically assess your solutions considering clinical, economic, and organisational impacts.
- Learn essential business skills, including project management, budgeting, intellectual property awareness, and scaling strategies.
- Test solutions on a smaller scale, adapt based on feedback, and continuously refine your approach.
- Consider how innovations will be maintained, funded, and integrated long-term into clinical practice.
- Clearly articulate the value and potential of your innovation, overcoming resistance by advocating for its necessity using data, not just moral arguments.
- Effective innovation often requires teamwork; focus on enabling the best solution, not necessarily doing everything yourself.

Reflective questions to consider to help you on your way to innovating in nursing

1 What outdated practices do I regularly encounter that could benefit from innovation?
2 Am I limiting my ideas based on current practices, or am I genuinely thinking creatively?
3 How comfortable am I with proposing solutions that might initially face resistance?

References

1   Rafferty, A. M., & Wall, B. (2010). An icon and iconoclast for today. In Nelson, S., & Rafferty, A. M. (Eds.), *Notes on Nightingale: The Influence and Legacy of a Nursing Icon* (p. 135). ILR Press.
2   Rabbitt, M. (2019). Modern-day Nightingales: Meet three enterprising nurses who moonlight as inventors. https://www.jnj.com/innovation/meet-3-nurses-who-moonlight-as-inventors-and-entrepreneurs

8   Harmonising compassion with critical thinking

Master the Balance of Heart and Head

Nightingale is typically remembered as the compassionate 'lady with the lamp', but contemporary observers saw something more formidable: a leader, strategist, and intellectual. Historians have long sought to challenge the one-dimensional portrayal of her legacy, a misconception that arguably continues to obscure the role of critical thinking and intellectual power in nursing today.

> It was inevitable under the circumstances, that an emotional interpretation should be given to the great work of rescue which Florence Nightingale accomplished, that heart should be put before head, and the 'commander of genius.' With her calm powers of organisation and discipline (subduing even blockheads and fools), should be hailed as an 'angel of mercy'... Had she been asked to choose her own motto, it would not have been 'blessed are the merciful'... by far more probably 'blessed are the masterful, for they shall obtain mastery'.[1]
>
> Laurence Houseman – The Great Victorians (1932)

Florence Nightingale is often remembered for her compassion, her famous nightly rounds with a lamp in hand, providing comfort to the wounded soldiers in the Crimean War. But what truly set her apart as a transformative figure in nursing was her ability to combine that compassion with sharp, critical thinking. Nightingale's unique blend of empathy and meticulous clinical reasoning allowed her to revolutionise healthcare, turning patient care into both an art and a science. Nightingale herself, in reference to her reputation as primarily of emotional or spiritual value as the 'lady with the lamp' allegedly described it as 'all that ministering angel nonsense'.[2] Nurses today can learn much from her example, as modern nursing requires not only emotional

DOI: 10.4324/9781003646259-9

intelligence but also the critical thinking necessary to navigate complex clinical environments and solve multifaceted health problems.

Nightingale's 'Lamp Rounds': compassion in action

Nightingale's rounds, often referred to as her 'lamp rounds', have become iconic in the history of nursing. She would walk the wards of the military hospital in Scutari at night, checking on each soldier by the light of a small lamp. These nightly rounds were more than a display of routine care; they symbolised her deep empathy and emotional support for the soldiers under her care. The soldiers, many of whom were far from home and suffering from severe injuries and illness, found comfort in Nightingale's presence. This display of compassion was not simply an emotional gesture. Nightingale understood the importance of holistic care, acknowledging not only the physical pain of her patients but also their emotional and psychological suffering. Modern nurses continue this tradition of providing emotional support to their patients, recognising that compassionate care leads to better patient outcomes, improved satisfaction, and a stronger nurse-patient relationship. However, compassion alone is not enough to address the complex healthcare challenges nurses face today. Nightingale's success lay in her ability to combine her empathy with critical thinking, ensuring that her patients not only felt supported but also received the highest standard of care which was the least likely to result in poor clinical outcomes.

Critical thinking: the foundation of Nightingale's success

While her lamp rounds are often romanticised, it was Nightingale's critical thinking that laid the foundation for her lasting influence on healthcare. Her work during the Crimean War was, as we have explored so far, driven by meticulous observation, data collection, and analysis. Nightingale's critical thinking allowed her to recognise that the root cause of these deaths was not primarily their battle injuries or inadequate medical treatment, but poor sanitation and ventilation. She systematically collected data on patient outcomes and hospital conditions, using this information to develop and implement hygiene protocols that drastically reduced mortality rates. Her approach, driven by *both* compassion for the suffering soldiers *and* a scientific, analytical mindset, led to reforms that saved countless lives. Compassion *alone*, sadly, does not save lives. Despite a focus on the compassionate components of nursing not being a core focus of Nightingales philosophy of nursing, a focus on caring was intensified in the 1970s with the publication of Jean Watsons Theory of Human Caring.[3] This theory very much emphasised the emotional features of nurses. On Watsons website in 2025 the following definition of 'caring science' is provided:

> Caring Science invites discovery and honoring of all the vicissitudes of
> humanity; honoring metaphysical phenomena such as Spirit, Sacred, Love,

Consciousness, and Caring (Caritas). Caring Science places nursing's phenomena within the Unitary Transformative paradigmatic thinking, accommodating phenomena such as non-local consciousness, transpersonal, transcendence, pattern, intentionality, sacred, and energy.[4]

Indeed, this more care-focused vision of nursing appears to have been adopted by the public. A 2022 study on public perceptions of nurses found that they are typically associated with emotional intelligence and compassion, while research skills and the integration of evidence into practice were seen as largely irrelevant.[5] The study also revealed that nurses are often perceived as lacking leadership capabilities. These are troubling findings. Beyond the reputational consequences, potentially undermining how seriously the profession is taken by the public, there are also significant conceptual critiques of 'care' as a foundational ethic for nursing.[6]

Foremost among these is the concept's vagueness. 'Caring' lacks a precise, universally accepted definition, rendering it an unstable foundation for a robust ethical or theoretical framework in nursing. For one nurse, caring might involve emotional availability; for another, technical excellence might be its highest expression. Consider Jean Watson's definition of caring, which includes notions such as 'accommodating non-local consciousness' and 'sacred energy', terms that are difficult to operationalise and subject to widely varying interpretations.

Additionally, a care-based ethic risks leading to exploitation of the caregiver, particularly in hierarchical or resource-poor systems. For example, a nurse who regularly works unpaid overtime out of a sense of duty to patients may inadvertently enable institutional exploitation, contributing to burnout and emotional exhaustion. Moreover, care ethics tend to be subjective, driven more by personal feelings than by consistent ethical principles. In complex situations, such as a disagreement between two nurses about whether to continue life-sustaining treatment, emotional attachments may override rational analysis, leading to unresolved ethical conflict.

Care ethics may also enable moral relativism, making it difficult to establish or apply universal standards. A nurse might provide more compassionate care to a patient who reminds them of a loved one, while unintentionally neglecting others. This emotional bias could lead to inconsistent care and feelings of neglect among other patients, with potential negative outcomes.

Furthermore, the emotional intensity associated with caring relationships may be psychologically unsustainable. A nurse who forms a deep attachment to a terminally ill patient may experience intense grief upon their death, impairing their ability to care for others and increasing the risk of compassion fatigue. In this way, caring, while virtuous, can become a liability in environments that require sustained resilience and clinical detachment.

A focus on the nurse's emotional labour may also obscure the patient's perspective. For instance, a nurse who resists using digital technologies out of concern for maintaining a 'human touch' may inadvertently deny patients tools that support autonomy, privacy, or independence.* Ironically, recent research suggests that patients may sometimes perceive artificial intelligence as more compassionate than human clinicians in emotionally challenging scenarios, even when unaware that the response was AI-generated.[†,7]

Finally, emotional involvement may compromise professional objectivity, a concern recognised in the guidance that healthcare professionals should avoid treating close family members. Emotional entanglement can impair clinical judgement, introducing risks that extend beyond the individual caregiver.

Compassion and critical thinking in modern nursing

Despite the numerous critiques of the concept of 'care', it is necessary to recognise its importance. No one wants an uncaring nurse if they can avoid it. The argument here is not that it is irrelevant, but that first, as Nightingale appeared to acknowledge – via omitting discussion of this issue in her writings or lectures, it is not an essential foundation for nursing. Second, an overemphasis on this issue appears to be cementing an image of nursing in the public mindset which denies its association with science, leadership and intellectual rigour. Unjust as this may feel, given the importance of empathy in all endeavours involving interpersonal communication, it seems that there is often a false dichotomy drawn between intellectualism and compassion. This is perhaps best reflected in the adage 'too posh to wash'[8] which is often used in arguments bemoaning the 'over-education' of nurses, which is suggested to somehow preclude them from basic compassion. These issues arguably have negative implications for patient care, recruitment of potential leaders into the profession, and salaries for nurses. Evidently, more economic value is placed on scientific and technical abilities, over perceived emotional capabilities. Nurses today, as every other health professional, are expected to exhibit both compassion and critical thinking in their daily practice. Compassion remains an important feature of nursing care, but critical thinking is equally, if not more, essential for solving complex clinical

---

* As Nightingale's contemporary, Sir William Osler, once said: '*There are individuals, doctors and nurses, for example, whose very existence is a constant reminder of our frailties.*' See Osler, W. (1904). *Aequanimitas, with Other Addresses to Medical Students, Nurses and Practitioners of Medicine.* HK Lewis.

† This is but one example, there is now an entire field of research on artificial empathy. Readers are strongly encouraged to explore this and form their own perspectives on its implications for nursing.

problems, making decisions in high-pressure environments, and ensuring patient safety.

Developing critical thinking skills in nursing

Critical thinking is an essential skill in nursing, cultivated through education, clinical experience, and reflective practice. Contemporary nursing education across many countries prioritises the development of critical thinking by teaching students to analyse complex information, apply evidence-based reasoning, and make sound clinical decisions. However, the ability to combine analytical thinking with compassion and holistic care comes not only from academic training but also from sustained clinical experience and a deep commitment to patient-centred practice.

Many modern nurses rightly express frustration at the fast-paced nature of today's clinical environments, which often leave little room for reflection or deep consideration of care. Yet this tension between task-oriented work and critical reflection is not new. Writing in 1874, Florence Nightingale highlighted a similar concern in a lecture to her nurses:

> So shall we do everything in our power to become proficient, not only in knowing the symptoms and what is to be done, but in knowing the "Reason Why" of such symptoms, and why such and such a thing is done; and so on, till we can some day train others to know the "reason why". Many say: "we have no time; the ward work gives us no time" But it is so easy to degenerate into a mere drudgery about the Wards, when we have goodwill to do it, and are fonder of practical work than of giving ourselves the trouble of learning the "reason why".[9]

Nightingale's words remind us that critical thinking is not merely a personal asset but a shared professional responsibility. By understanding the 'why' behind nursing actions, nurses become better equipped not only to improve care but also to educate others. Unfortunately, many aspects of nursing still suffer from unanswered 'why' questions. For example, despite decades of research, the prevention of pressure injuries (then termed 'bed sores' by Nightingale) remains a complex issue with major gaps in the evidence base.[10] Likewise, the control of communicable diseases continues to challenge healthcare systems. In fact, a whole specialty, infection prevention nursing, emerged in the 1950s to combat hospital-acquired infections and rising antibiotic resistance, problems that have only intensified with time.[11]

There remains a pressing need for nurses who are not only doers but also thinkers, professionals who seek to answer the unanswered and push the boundaries of nursing knowledge. As Nightingale urged, we must make time for inquiry, for learning the 'reason why,' and for sharing that knowledge with others.

Key lessons for modern nurses to achieve the Nightingale Effect

- Balance emotion with reason. Nightingale's power came not just from her compassion, but from her disciplined, scientific mindset. Modern nurses must carry forward both heartfelt care and rigorous, evidence-based practice.
- Challenge the stereotypes. The image of the nurse as solely compassionate or subservient undermines the intellectual demands of the role. Nurses must reclaim their identity as clinical thinkers, researchers, and leaders.
- Ask the 'reason why'. Nightingale urged nurses to understand the rationale behind every action. This mindset still matters, pushing nurses beyond task-based work into reflective, analytical practice.
- Don't dismiss the emotional self, but don't be governed by it. Compassion is vital, but over-identification with suffering can blur judgement. Emotional intelligence should be paired with ethical clarity and professional distance.
- Be a force for intellectual growth in others. Critical thinking is not only for individual benefit. Just as Nightingale envisioned, nurses must foster knowledge and reflection in others through mentorship, research, and teaching.

Some reflective questions to consider to help you find balance between heart and head

1 What 'why' questions remain unanswered in your clinical area and what could be done about these?
2 When was the last time you questioned a routine task and sought to understand the reasoning behind it?
3 Have you ever felt pressure to downplay your critical thinking in favour of being seen as 'caring'? How did you respond?

References

1 Houseman in Massingham, H. J., & Massingham, H. (1937). *The Great Victorians* (p. 364). Penguin Books. https://14.139.58.199:8080/jspui/handle/123456789/2319
2 Bostridge, M. (2008). *Florence Nightingale: The Woman and Her Legend* (p. 502). Penguin.
3 Watson, J. (1997). The theory of human caring: Retrospective and prospective. *Nursing Science Quarterly*, 10(1), 49–52. https://doi.org/10.1177/089431849701000114
4 Jean Watson Caring Science Theory. https://www.watsoncaringscience.org/jean-bio/caring-science-theory/#theory – accessed March 2025.

5 Rodríguez-Pérez, M., Mena-Navarro, F., Domínguez-Pichardo, A., & Teresa-Morales, C. (2022). Current social perception of and value attached to nursing professionals' competences: An integrative review. *International Journal of Environmental Research and Public Health*, 19(3), 1817. https://doi.org/10.3390/ijerph19031817

6 Crigger, N. J. (1997). The trouble with caring: A review of eight arguments against an ethic of care. *Journal of Professional Nursing*, 13(4), 217–221. https://doi.org/10.1016/S8755-7223(97)80091-9

7 Ovsyannikova, D., de Mello, V. O., & Inzlicht, M. (2025). Third-party evaluators perceive AI as more compassionate than expert humans. *Communications Psychology*, 3, 4. https://doi.org/10.1038/s44271-024-00182-6

8 Oliver, D. (2017). David Oliver: why shouldn't nurses be graduates? *BMJ*, 356, j863. https://doi.org/10.1136/bmj.j863

9 Nightingale, F. (1915). *Nightingale to Her Nurses* (p. 70). Macmillan and Co.

10 National Pressure Injury Advisory Panel, European Pressure Ulcer Advisory Panel, & Pan Pacific Pressure Injury Alliance. (2025). *Prevention and Treatment of Pressure Ulcers/Injuries: Clinical Practice Guideline* (Fourth Edition). Emily Haesler (Ed.). [Cited: 06/05/2025]. https://internationalguideline.com

11 Torriani, F., & Taplitz, R. (2010). History of infection prevention and control. In Jonathan Cohen, Steven M. Opal and William G. (Eds.), *Infectious Diseases* (pp. 76–85). Mosby. https://doi.org/10.1016/B978-0-323-04579-7.00006-X

9 Mentoring and inspiring future leaders

Sow Seeds of Greatness in Others

> *True mentorship is not about hierarchy or replication, it is about recognising potential, learning together, and encouraging others to go further than we ever could. Linda Richards, one of Nightingale's most notable mentees, captured this philosophy perfectly in her memoirs.*
>
> True progress in the largest sense comes most rapidly by acknowledging good work wherever it is found, and by learning to follow the good example.[1]
>
> Linda Richards 1911

During a pouring rainstorm, one morning in the middle of August 1877, a young American nurse named Linda Richards arrived in London with a dream. She had crossed the Atlantic for one purpose: to learn from the legendary Florence Nightingale. Having already sought nursing training in Boston after a pattern established by the Deaconesses at Kaiserworth* she was left disillusioned, describing the nurses she worked with as *'thoughtless, careless, and often heartless'*.[1] Inspired by reading a book written by a former student of Nightingales at St Thomas's Hospital, she decided that to achieve a proper nurse training she had to study at the source.

At the time, Nightingale was elderly and often confined to her home, her health long diminished by the effects of her service during the Crimean War. Richards was granted the rare privilege of studying at St. Thomas' Hospital, home of the Nightingale Training School. Though they would not meet often in person, Nightingale sent Richards letters. Nightingale's mentorship wasn't loud or performative. It was written in ink, steeped in purpose, and always aimed at empowering others to go further.

---

* This was also where Nightingale obtained her first nursing experiences.

DOI: 10.4324/9781003646259-10

In a letter to the matron of the Royal Infirmary in Edinburgh, Nightingale shared her reflections on Richards:

A Miss Richards, a Boston lady, training matron to the Massachusetts General Hospital, has in a very spirited manner come to us for training to herself... I have seldom seen anyone who struck me as so admirable. I think we have as much to learn from her as she from us.[1]

This candid observation reflects a surprising humility and mutuality. While Richards approached the encounter with awe, '*Even now I can distinctly recall with what fear and trembling I walked toward the house...*'.[1] Nightingale framed the relationship as reciprocal. She actively engaged with Richards' experience of American nursing, demonstrating sincere curiosity about transatlantic differences in practice. As Richards recalled, '*Miss Nightingale showed the truest interest in our American training schools*'.[1]

On Richards' departure, Nightingale offered a parting hope, not of replication, but of transcendence: '*May you outstrip us, that we in turn may outstrip you*'.[1]

Richards did just that. She went on to establish training schools across the United States and Japan, becoming widely recognised as America's first professionally trained nurse. Her legacy was not simply an extension of Nightingale's, it was a flowering of it.

Nightingale's legacy in nursing education

The story of Linda Richards is but one example of many individuals who Nightingale personally impacted through her efforts to improve nursing. In 1860, she founded the Nightingale School of Nursing at St. Thomas' Hospital in London, the first professional nursing school in the world. This marked the beginning of a formalised nursing education system, moving nursing from a role often viewed as domestic or informal into a recognised, respected profession with specific training and standards. Nightingale's vision for her school was not just to train nurses in technical skills but to imbue them with the ethical principles, compassion, and critical thinking skills that she believed were essential to excellent patient care. Nightingale understood that nursing education didn't stop with the acquisition of basic skills; it required continuous learning, growth, and the development of leadership qualities. As she said during a lecture in 1872:

A woman who thinks in herself: "Now I am a 'full' Nurse a 'skilled' Nurse, I have learnt all that there is to be learnt": take my word for it, she does not know what a Nurse is, and she never will know; she is gone back already. Conceit and Nursing cannot exist in the same person[2]

Nightingale – Lecture to her nurses 1872

The example set by Nightingale reflects contemporary studies on the experiences and perspectives in relation to mentorship. In a recent Norwegian study, practising nurses reported that wanting to be an example and role model and flexibility to new knowledge were both considered to be important factors in effective mentorship.[3] In another study, participants reported that time spent with a mentor does not necessarily impact the perceptions of value, instead genuineness and respect are perceived to be of greater importance.[4] These were both qualities it seems Richards found in Nightingale.

Reflections on mentorship

The story of Florence Nightingale and Linda Richards challenges us to reframe mentorship as a shared journey rather than a one-way exchange. While Richards approached Nightingale with awe, it was Nightingale who insisted that she, too, had something to learn. This quiet, radical humility is at the heart of great mentorship: it is not about hierarchy, but about shared purpose and mutual growth.

Today, the best mentors do more than teach, they learn, adapt, and listen. In the fast-evolving landscape of healthcare, mentorship is not simply about passing down techniques, but about nurturing character, modelling ethical practice, and fostering the courage to lead. As research highlights, being a role model and remaining open to new knowledge are essential traits of effective mentors. It reminds us that the power of mentorship lies not in the quantity of time spent, but in the quality of the connection, marked by respect, authenticity, and belief in the other's potential. Much of mentorship takes place in the invisible curriculum: the handwritten feedback, the quiet encouragement, the wordless affirmation that someone believes in your future. Mentorship is as much about shaping identity as it is about shaping skill. In this way, the act becomes legacy.

Perhaps the most profound mentoring statement Nightingale made was not instructional but aspirational: '*May you outstrip us, that we in turn may outstrip you*'. It reframes mentorship not as control, but as generative hope, a desire to see others go further, and in doing so, to raise the standard for all.

To mentor, then, is to plant seeds you may never see bloom, trusting that the garden will one day be more vibrant because you chose to sow.

Key lessons for modern nurses to achieve the Nightingale Effect

- Mentorship is mutual, it isn't a top-down transfer of knowledge or skill, but a reciprocal relationship rooted in humility. Great nurses remain open to the wisdom of others, regardless of age, title, or origin.
- Aim for empowerment over instructions. Support others to grow in confidence and capability, rather than create dependency.
- Lead quietly but with purpose Nightingales letters were quiet acts of leadership. The modern nurse can lead through quiet integrity, by example and through encouragement.
- Legacy is built through others. The Nightingale Effect can be measured by how far those we mentor can go. Mentorship should aim to elevate others beyond our own accomplishments, recognising that progress is a shared endeavour.
- Mentorship is grounded in mutual respect, not status or authority. As research shows, genuine connection is more powerful than time spent together.

Reflective questions to consider to help you to provide better mentorship

1 What was the most valuable experience I had with a mentor as a student or junior nurse?
2 How open am I to learning from those with less experience and professional status than myself?
3 How do you offer feedback and encouragement? Are there opportunities to be more intentional in supporting others' growth?

References

1 Richards, L. (1911). *Reminiscences of Linda Richards: America's First Trained Nurse* (pp. 18, 22, 37, 52, 53, 116). https://archive.org/details/reminiscencesofl00rich/page/120/mode/2up?q=trembling
2 Nightingale, F. (1915). *Nightingale to Her Nurses* (p. 1). Macmillan and Co.
3 Kallerhult Hermansson, S., Kasén, A., Hilli, Y., Norström, F., Vaag, J. R., & Bölenius, K. (2024). Exploring registered nurses' perspectives as mentors for newly qualified nurses: A qualitative interview study. *BMJ Open*, 14(5), e082940. https://doi.org/10.1136/bmjopen-2023-082940
4 Baxter, G., & McGowan, B. (2022). An exploration of undergraduate nursing students' experiences of mentorship in an Irish hospital. *British Journal of Nursing (Mark Allen Publishing)*, 31(15), 812–817. https://doi.org/10.12968/bjon.2022.31.15.812

10 Challenging norms to drive healthcare innovation

Break the Chains of Tradition

> *Progress cannot result from complacency. Nightingale's entire career was driven by a refusal to accept what was, socially, professionally, and intellectually. Her work reflects a call to reclaim that discontent as a generative force for change.*
>
> Were there none who were discontented with what they have, the world would never reach anything better.[1]
>
> Florence Nightingale, Cassandra

Florence Nightingale's revolutionary impact on nursing and public health would have been impossible had she accepted the conventional wisdom of her time. Born into a wealthy British family in 1820, Nightingale was groomed for a life of comfort, domesticity, and social propriety. A woman of her social standing was expected to marry advantageously and serve as the moral and managerial centre of the household. Nursing, by contrast, was perceived as a lowly occupation, grubby, physically taxing, and morally suspect. Yet, in an act of radical defiance, Nightingale rejected this preordained path and embraced a calling that would redefine healthcare. By stepping beyond societal expectations, Nightingale not only redefined what it meant to be a nurse, she also expanded what it meant to be a woman with agency in a rigidly patriarchal society. In doing so, she opened a space for future nurses to challenge other ingrained norms, for example, those of race, gender, and hierarchy. Today's nurses inherit this legacy of disruption and reinvention, with the power to question outdated assumptions and reimagine healthcare delivery in bold and transformative ways.

But Nightingale's contribution was not merely one of social rebellion, it was also epistemological. Her book '*Notes on Nursing: What It Is and What It Is Not*' remains foundational in nursing history, yet it offers no definitive

DOI: 10.4324/9781003646259-11

description of what nursing actually *is* (ironically). This omission, far from being a flaw, may be among Nightingale's most profound insights. Rather than pinning nursing down within rigid conceptual boundaries, she left room for the profession to define, and redefine, itself across time and context. This may have been in recognition that the liberties attached to women's professional activities may well change over time. In this ambiguity lies a powerful invitation. Rather than limiting the scope of the profession, the vagueness surrounding nursing's essence can be seen as liberating. It encourages nurses to engage critically and creatively with the question of what nursing is and what it could become. It challenges each generation to construct its own conception of the nursing mission in light of the paradigmatic shifts in science, technology, society, and patient needs. Indeed, Nightingale's reluctance to strictly categorise nursing might seem destabilising, perhaps even undermining to the project of professionalisation. Yet this openness may be precisely what enables nursing to remain agile in the face of emerging crises. Whether it is the global burden of chronic disease, pandemics, digital transformation, or health inequities, the ability of nursing to adapt, reform, and resist ossification is a direct result of its philosophical malleability. Contemporary nursing philosophers have highlighted the issues that trying to force conformity into the practice of nursing has, typically resulting in rigid competency frameworks, and in some cases mandated engagement with seemingly arbitrary licensing and regulatory processes. This has been described as reflective primarily of an effort by the nursing profession to gain power and prestige for the discipline, potentially at the cost of attention on improving health outcomes.[2] It seems probable that Nightingale would have to some extent, agreed with these reflections. She was notably resistant to the notion of nurses having a professional register due to its potential to hinder the growth of the profession and exclude working-class women who typically had lower literacy abilities. These issues of the nature and purpose of the professionalisation of nursing are worthy of reflection by all nurses. No clear answer will be provided here as to what is best for the profession, however, the lack of a unifying theory of nursing practice or clear epistemology remain 'social facts' about the profession itself. What to do about this is up to nurses themselves. Since Nightingale, efforts have been made to provide clarity on what the rightful domain of nursing should be, these most notably include Fawcett's nursing metaparadigm.[3] The metaparadigm was intended to guide research and in theory, practice. Fawcett systematically synthesised the numerous nursing theories available at the time to identify the key concepts which are unique to the discipline. These, it was argued, included 'the person', 'the environment', 'health', and 'nursing practice'. The obvious issue with this, however, is that 'nursing practice' cannot define itself solely by referencing its own domain, it becomes a circular proposition. Without anchoring these concepts in a broader epistemological or ontological framework, they risk becoming abstract ideals rather than operational foundations. In this light, the metaparadigm serves more as a heuristic tool than a definitive structure.

Moreover, the absence of a unifying epistemology invites continued ambiguity about what nurses do, know, and ought to know. This ambiguity may create space for innovation, but it also renders the profession vulnerable to external definitions imposed by medical professionals, policy, or technology, often with little reference to nurses' knowledge or interests. The future of nursing's identity therefore lies not in settling once and for all what nursing 'is', but in fostering a profession-wide capacity to reflexively interrogate its purposes, limits, and potential. The question is not simply what should define nursing, but *who* should define it, and under what conditions. Reclaiming that authority may be the most critical task of all. This no simple task, however. Efforts to re-assert professional status and establish scientific authority have been sought via attempts to change the semantics surrounding the naming of the profession. This has resulted in the promotion of the use of the term 'nursology' by some nurse theorists, to describe a unique 'nursing science'.* However, it has also been pointed out that this playing with semantics makes no meaningful change to the knowledge nurses hold or has any material impact on the nature of the discipline in any real way which affects nursing goals or outcomes.[4]

While Nightingale evidently grappled with the problem of 'what nursing is', she did not seek to enforce her own rigid rules as to what nurses should and shouldn't be doing. Her philosophy was clearly motivated more by her fundamental beliefs in the dignity of humanity, and highly responsive to the particular challenges she observed in the world at the time she was working. She was unconcerned by the status of nursing, if she had been it seems probable, she would not have entered the profession to begin with. What concerned her was the health and wellbeing of her fellow humans. The methods, skills, knowledge, and collaborators she needed to achieve this more fundamental goal were always secondary to the ethical imperative that underpinned her work. Nightingale's flexibility, her capacity to borrow from science, theology, statistics, architecture, and philosophy, reveals a model of nursing grounded not in rigid disciplinary boundaries, but in a deep responsiveness to suffering and need.

This responsiveness is what makes her legacy worthy of continued reflection. It offers an important counterpoint to modern efforts to codify and professionalise nursing in ways that risk prioritising form over function, and status over service. Rather than seeking legitimacy through mimicry of medicine or theoretical abstraction, Nightingale reminds us that the heart of nursing lies in its relational, context-sensitive, and moral commitments.

In the current age of digital transformation and policy-driven practice, this ethos remains more vital than ever. Nurses must ask not only how to define their work, but how to preserve the freedom and responsibility to define it on their own terms, in alignment with the needs of the people they care for, rather than the imperatives of the systems they work within.

---

*   There is an entire website dedicated to this concept – https://nursology.net/

Key challenges in modern healthcare

In our era, where healthcare faces mounting pressures and rapid change however, the ongoing epistemic indeterminacy becomes a site of potential rather than weakness. Future nurses, in embracing the unresolved nature of their craft, are not abandoning professionalism, they are advancing it. Like Nightingale, they are called not to replicate norms, but to reshape them. To be discontented with what is, in order to imagine and build what might be.

Examples of the key challenges faced by modern healthcare systems include the rapid advancement of artificial intelligence technologies and the associated development of big data in healthcare, globalisation, climate change, pandemic disease, global ageing, and antimicrobial resistance. In addition to these, cultural shifts including the increasing predominance of social media as a means to form human connections have created very different dynamics between nurses and their patients. As one of my former undergraduate students once pertinently stated, *'our patients are online now, we need to meet them there'*. Other areas of technological change have seen the increase in the interest and use of robotics in nursing care.[†] Despite these potentially transformative impacts of modern technologies, a recent report on the UK National Health System described it as *'in the foothills of digital transformation'*,[5] with digital data stored within the system seldom exploited for its potential research benefits. This clearly indicates a great deal of low hanging fruit, ready to be harvested by nurses with Nightingalean curiosity and drive to improve healthcare.

Reclaiming the future of nursing

The legacy of Florence Nightingale reminds us that the strength of nursing lies not in rigid definitions or institutional prestige, but in a deeply ethical responsiveness to the needs of humanity. In a time of enormous social, technological, and environmental upheaval, nurses are again called to challenge norms and reimagine what care looks like in a changing world. The very ambiguity that once frustrated efforts to categorise nursing now reveals itself as a powerful resource: a space of creative, ethical, and intellectual freedom. Rather than passively absorbing externally imposed roles, from artificial intelligence to institutional performance metrics, nurses can and must *shape* these forces in alignment with the profession's enduring values. Nightingale's refusal to be constrained by her era's expectations must now become our refusal to be defined by the external influences on the profession's development. To break the chains of tradition is not to reject all that has come before, but to remain

---

† For an early text dedicated to this issue see – Tanioka, T., Yasuhara, Y., Osaka, K., Ito, H., & Locsin, R. C. (Eds.). (2023). *Nursing Robots and Robotics in Nursing: Robotic Technology and Human Caring*. Independently Published. ISBN: 979-8398280159

alert to when those traditions no longer serve the good. It is to refuse silence in the face of injustice, to embrace epistemic humility without losing professional courage, and to take seriously the ethical imperative to care, not as a function, but as a philosophy.

Let us then be discontented, not as a posture of complaint, but as a commitment to transformation. For it is in this spirit of reflective resistance, of principled reinvention, that the true future of nursing, and the health of the communities it serves will be secured.

Key lessons for modern nurses to achieve the Nightingale Effect

- Discontent is not a flaw; it is a signal that change is necessary. Like Nightingale, modern nurses should see dissatisfaction as the starting point for innovation and ethical transformation.
- The goal is not to elevate nursing for its own sake, but to improve lives. Tradition should be respected but not revered when it obstructs progress or care.
- Nursing does not need rigid definitions to be strong. Its strength lies in its capacity to adapt, redefine itself, and respond ethically to human need.
- The lack of a fixed epistemology in nursing isn't a weakness but a space for philosophical and practical freedom. It invites every nurse to think critically about what nursing should be, in their time and place.
- Nightingale acted not for the profession's honour, but for human dignity. Today's nurses should guard against professionalisation efforts that erode the relational and ethical heart of care.
- From AI and robotics to global pandemics, nurses must shape the forces acting upon them. Do not be passive recipients, be active authors of the profession's evolution.

Some reflective questions to consider to help you break the chains of conventionality in nursing:

1 What is the most useful thing I could do for my patients which I am not currently doing?
2 What societal or professional expectations have I internalised about nursing, and how might these limit my ability to provide the best care?
3 Do I feel empowered to help define what nursing is in my context, or am I waiting (or currently relying) on someone else to define it for me?

References

1 Nightingale, F. (1979 [1852]). *Cassandra* (p. 29). Old Westbury. https://archive.org/details/cassandraessay0000nigh/page/28/mode/2up?q=discontented
2 Drevdahl, D. J., & Canales, M. K. (2023). Nursing's endless pursuit of professionalization. In Martin Lipscomb (Ed.), *Routledge Handbook of Philosophy and Nursing* (pp. 215–226). Routledge. https://doi.org/10.4324/9781003427407-26
3 Fawcett, J. (1984). The metaparadigm of nursing: Present status and future refinements. *Image: The Journal of Nursing Scholarship*, 16(3), 84–87. https://doi.org/10.1111/j.1547-5069.1984.tb01393.x
4 Parse, R. R. (2019). Nursology: What's in a name? *Nursing Science Quarterly*, 32(2), 93–94. https://doi.org/10.1177/0894318419831619
5 Darzi, A. (2024). *Independent Investigation of the National Health Service in England* (p. 8). Department of Health and Social Care. https://assets.publishing.service.gov.uk/media/66f42ae630536cb92748271f/Lord-Darzi-Independent-Investigation-of-the-National-Health-Service-in-England-Updated-25-September.pdf

Conclusion

Towards a Nightingalean model of nursing leadership

> *In* Cassandra, *Nightingale articulates a profound truth about leadership and progress: that meaningful change often demands struggle, discomfort, and even personal sacrifice. Her words challenge us to understand that suffering is not always a sign of failure, but a necessary consequence of pushing boundaries. A Nightingalean model of nursing leadership must therefore be grounded in moral purpose, intellectual courage, and a willingness to act despite adversity.*
>
> ...out of suffering may come the cure. Better have pain than paralysis! A hundred struggle and drown in the breakers. One discovers the new world. But rather, ten times rather, die in the surf, heralding the way to that new world, than stand idly on the shore![1]
>
> Florence Nightingale – Cassandra

Florence Nightingale's greatness as a nurse didn't stem solely from her bedside care; it was her ability to see the bigger picture and advocate for systemic change via her writing, lectures, letters, and political lobbying that set her apart. Today's nurses have the same opportunity to drive institutional reforms that improve patient outcomes on a large scale. Greatness in nursing is not about being perfect or working in ideal conditions. It is about making a difference in small, meaningful ways, even when faced with systemic challenges and personal limitations.

In today's fast-paced and often under-resourced healthcare environments, striving for greatness can seem overwhelming or even unattainable. The increasing demands on nurses, due to higher patient loads, administrative burdens, and technological pressures, often leave little room for the type of work that Nightingale championed. Yet, it is in these very moments of strain that the pursuit of nursing greatness becomes even more critical. The risks of not striving for greatness and maintaining a focus on our patients and our own

DOI: 10.4324/9781003646259-12

development were also recognised well by Nightingale: '*The world, more especially the Hospital world, is in such a hurry, is moving so fast, that it is too easy to slide into bad habits before we are aware*'.[2]

Nurses today face challenges that Nightingale herself could never have imagined, from the complexities of global pandemics to the rapid integration of AI and digital health technologies. But the core principles of nursing, empathy, advocacy, and an unwavering commitment to patient well-being, remain unchanged. This message is as relevant to today's nurses as it was in Nightingale's time. The structural challenges that persist in healthcare, understaffing, bureaucratic red tape, resource shortages, can make it feel as though striving for greatness is out of reach. But the key is not to focus on what can't be changed immediately, but rather on the incremental changes we can make, one patient, one shift, one advocacy effort at a time. It is normal to feel that change is slow, challenging and that the work of a single nurse is limited. At the end of her reminiscences, Linda Richards, one of Nightingales most significant students, humbly concludes:

As for my own work, I often feel that, for the many years I have served, I have accomplished little. Whether I have been a wise builder, someone else must decide. All I can say is that I have found life full of interest in an earnest endeavor to do faithfully my small part in the great movement which has resulted in establishing the profession of the trained nurse in America.[3]

Nurses who consistently push for improvement, despite the limitations of the system, are the ones who make lasting changes that echo throughout their institutions and communities. It is easy to get trapped in a cycle of evaluating the magnitude of one's contribution, without paying sufficient attention to its value to those whom it may affect. It is important not to lose sight of this. As Nightingale put it:

My patients are watching me: They know what my profession, my calling is: to devote myself to the good of the sick. They are asking themselves: does that nurse act up to her profession? This is no supposition. It is a fact. It is a call to us, to each individual nurse, to act up to her profession.[2]

As you reflect on the strategies and lessons from Florence Nightingale's life, remember that the path to nursing greatness is not a single moment of triumph but a lifetime of persistence, learning, and leadership. By continuing to strive for excellence, even in the smallest acts of care, and by advocating for the changes that will improve patient outcomes and the profession as a whole, you contribute to the enduring legacy of nursing greatness. The world needs great nurses now more than ever, those who will challenge the status quo, push for better systems, and ultimately improve the health and well-being of those they serve. Greatness in nursing is not about what we accomplish alone, but about how we lift up the entire profession by improving care for patients, advocating for those who cannot advocate for themselves, and inspiring the next generation of nurses. The pursuit of greatness is ongoing, and each nurse has the opportunity to make a profound impact.

The Nightingale Effect: A description of nursing greatness

To embody the Nightingale Effect is to embrace nursing not as a fixed role, but as a dynamic, ethical force for human good. Nursing greatness is not found in status, formal authority, compliance, or tradition for its own sake, but in the courageous pursuit of better care, even when it disrupts convention. It is in questioning what has always been done, resisting superficial profes- sionalisation, and defining practice through purpose rather than prescription. Nightingale's legacy teaches us that greatness lies in balancing compassion with intellect, leadership with humility, and tradition with innovation. Today's great nurses are system-changers, silent mentors, critical thinkers, and bold advocates who are not content to be passive cogs in a broken machine. They question, create, and connect. They listen to discontent as the first whisper of change. The Nightingale Effect is not a destination; it is a way of seeing, thinking, and acting, an ongoing commitment to lead by light, innovate with care, and serve with both head and heart.

References

1 Nightingale, F. (1979 [1852]). *Cassandra* (p. 29). Old Westbury. https://archive.org/ details/cassandraessay0000nigh/page/28/mode/2up?q=discontented
2 Nightingale, F. (1915). *Nightingale to Her Nurses* (pp. 49, 143). Macmillan and Co.
3 Richards, L. (1911). *Reminiscences of Linda Richards: America's First Trained Nurse* (p. 117). Lippincott. https://archive.org/details/reminiscencesofl00rich/page/ 120/mode/2up?q=trembling

Afterword

It is not easy to capture in words the enduring power of a life like Florence Nightingale's. Across this book, I have attempted to consider not only her extraordinary accomplishments but also the qualities of spirit, intellect, and discipline that made her one of the most transformative figures in the history of nursing. Nightingale is not just a nursing icon, she was a strategist, a reformer, and a quiet revolutionary. Her work was rooted in rigorous thinking, compassion, and a relentless pursuit of excellence. And yet, even in her own time, she became more than a person, she became a symbol of light in darkness. The poet Henry Wadsworth Longfellow, though never having met her, understood this deeply. His poem *Santa Filomena*, written in 1857, helped cement the image of Nightingale as 'The Lady with the Lamp', moving silently among the wounded, bringing hope and healing where others brought only war and despair. This image is not just a romantic embellishment, it captures something real and vital about Nightingale's legacy: her presence. Not just physical presence, but moral presence, intellectual presence, and the enduring light of her influence, which continues to guide nurses and carers across the world.

As we consider what it means to be great in nursing *today*, and as we strive to live out the principles Nightingale exemplified, advocacy, precision, courage, and humility, it seems fitting to let Longfellow's words remind us of how deeply the world felt her impact.

Here, in its entirety, is *Santa Filomena*, a poetic tribute to a woman whose light has never gone out.

Santa Filomena
By Henry Wadsworth Longfellow

Whene'er a noble deed is wrought,
Whene'er is spoken a noble thought,
Our hearts, in glad surprise,
To higher levels rise.

The tidal wave of deeper souls
Into our inmost being rolls,
And lifts us unawares
Out of all meaner cares.

Honor to those whose words or deeds
Thus help us in our daily needs,
And by their overflow
Raise us from what is low!

Thus thought I, as by night I read
Of the great army of the dead,
The trenches cold and damp,
The starved and frozen camp,

The wounded from the battle-plain,
In dreary hospitals of pain,
The cheerless corridors,
The cold and stony floors.

Lo! in that house of misery
A lady with a lamp I see
Pass through the glimmering gloom,
And flit from room to room.

And slow, as in a dream of bliss,
The speechless sufferer turns to kiss
Her shadow, as it falls
Upon the darkening walls.

As if a door in heaven should be
Opened, and then closed suddenly,
The vision came and went,
The light shone and was spent.

On England's annals, through the long
Hereafter of her speech and song,
That light its rays shall cast
From portals of the past.

A Lady with a Lamp shall stand
In the great history of the land,
A noble type of good,
Heroic womanhood.

Nor even shall be wanting here
The palm, the lily, and the spear,
The symbols that of yore
Saint Filomena bore.

I hope this poem serves as an invitation and inspiration to all who read this
book and feel called to follow in Nightingale's footsteps, not in imitation, but
in spirit. Her work is not finished. Her lamp still burns.

Further reading and resources

Key works by Nightingale (These texts are freely available online as they are now out of copyright)

- *Notes on Nursing*
- *Notes on Hospitals*
- *Nightingale to Her Nurses*

Biographical works on Nightingale

- Mark Bostridge, *Florence Nightingale: The Woman and Her Legend*. Penguin.
- Lynn McDonnald (editor), *The Collected Works of Florence Nightingale*. https://cwfn.uoguelph.ca/ (This is the most extensive collection of Nightingale's work currently available and may serve as a rich resource to those undertaking research into Nightingale's life and work).
- Lynn McDonald, *Florence Nightingale, Nursing and Health Care Today*. Springer.
- Sioban Nelson and Anne Marrie Rafferty (editors), *Notes on Nightingale: The Influence and Legacy of a Nursing Icon*. Cornell University Press.

Innovation in nursing

- FutureNurse. https://futurenurse.uk/
- National Health Service – Clinical Entrepreneur Programme. https://www.england.nhs.uk/aac/what-we-do/how-can-the-aac-help-me/clinical-entrepreneur-programme/
- National Health Service – Innovation Service. https://innovation.nhs.uk/

Research in nursing

- Contact your local hospital/service research department who may support you to develop ideas for research in practice.
- Contact local academics involved in the field of research you are interested in; they are likely to provide support and guidance to support your projects.

Organisations who support nurses to develop leadership skills

- The Florence Nightingale Foundation. https://florence-nightingale-foundation.org.uk/
- NursingNow. https://www.nursingnow.org/about/
- The National Health Service Leadership Academy. https://www.leadershipacademy.nhs.uk/
- Sigma Nursing (Global) – Provides leadership, research, and mentorship resources for nurses worldwide. https://www.sigmanursing.org/

Professional nursing organisations

- International Council of Nurses. https://www.icn.ch/

Index

Note: **Bold** page numbers refer to tables, *italic* page numbers refer to figures.

For Product Safety Concerns and Information please contact our EU
representative GPSR@taylorandfrancis.com
Taylor & Francis Verlag GmbH, Kaufingerstraße 24, 80331 München, Germany